I0026967

The Secrets of Modern Medicine Revealed

www.medicinerevealed.com

The Secrets of Modern Medicine Revealed

www.medicinerevealed.com

The Secrets of Modern Medicine Revealed

A journey into the secret world of modern medical practice as seen from the eye of the doctor

www.medicinerevealed.com

MedTale Publishing
Omaha, Nebraska

www.medicinerevealed.com

The Secrets of Modern Medicine Revealed

Manufactured in the USA

MedTale Publishing

Omaha, NE

Specializing in books of general interest related to medicine

Disclaimer: The information presented in this book and the website is meant to give general readers an interesting inside information about how modern medicine is practiced. All ideas expressed are the author's opinion and should not be, in any way, taken as medical advice. You should consult with your own doctor if you need any specific advice about your medical problems.

Library of Congress Control Number: 2010903954

ISBN-13: 978-0-9826965-0-7

ISBN-10: 0982696507

www.medicinerevealed.com

Welcome to the world of modern medical practice.

www.medicinerevealed.com

The Secrets of Modern Medicine Revealed

www.medicinerevealed.com

Dedicated to all my patients and their loved ones

www.medicinerevealed.com

The Secrets of Modern Medicine Revealed

www.medicinerevealed.com

Table of Contents

Chapter 1: Introduction

There is so much mystic, magic and miracle associated with the profession of medicine that it is every father's dream to see his child grow up to become a doctor — a person with the power to heal and save lives. Most future doctors are initially drawn to pursue a career in this noble profession with this vision of the healer in mind. They all want to become this great person who, with the knowledge and power gained from the medical school, is able to save lives and make a person smile by taking away the pain and suffering. But the road that leads to the ultimate destiny of becoming the healer is long and complex. The bars are high and the threshold to even commit to pursue this profession is so high that you need a very high degree of determination to pursue the path. Those who are lucky enough to get high grades, impressive resume and excellent source of financing get into medical school after a lot of hard work.

> After years of medical training, the doctor becomes so much absorbed in the technical details of the medical science that the words "healing" and "relieve suffering" do not make any sense to him and are soon replaced by "tissue regeneration" and "pain control".

After they finally get into medical school, something changes. They slowly start to lose the glamorous vision of medical career and start to struggle with the day-to-day technicalities of their course material. With today's advanced medical technology, their learning material becomes so much detailed in scientific description that they even tend to forget that the main objective of their study is to help humans. They become so obsessed with the details of bones, muscles, blood and body chemicals that they start looking at human body as something of a materialistic object that can be described in terms of the components that it is made up of. By the time they are done with the first half of their course, they have acquired extensive knowledge about how human body works and how each organ functions. It seems to them as if the whole person suddenly disappears and is replaced by an assembly of working parts, each with a distinct function.

Later on when they actually start seeing real patients, they will be reminded of the ultimate objective of their study. But, by that time, they have been so bugged down with the details of factual knowledge and scientific explanations that they no longer see, feel or perceive the romantic, magical, mystic or divine nature of their profession. By this time the words “human suffering”, “touching”, “protecting”, the same words that drew them to pursue this profession, seem awkwardly foreign and meaningless to them. Instead, they are now mainly concerned with “diagnosis”, “disease process”, “surgical procedure” and “drug interaction”. Now, they do not speak of healing, but talk about tissue regeneration instead. Now, they do not talk about relieving human suffering but talk about pain control and anesthesia. They do not talk about sadness or misery but talk about depression instead. Now they do not talk about magical touch but talk about detailed physical exam, x-rays and CAT scans.

When they actually start their medical practice after years of training, they eventually realize that they are dealing with human beings with emotions, expectations, wants, needs and curiosity. But they quickly adapt to this new discovery and develop two different types of languages and communication skills — first one to deal with other physicians or health care providers and a second one to deal with patients and their family. They try their best to explain the findings, disease process and treatment modalities to the patients in so called layman terms. But they feel that there is always a limit as to how much they can explain in this way and how much really needs to be explained.

The impact of medical profession is very profound on the society. Even a simple advice from the doctor has a long lasting impression on any family. We have all grown up with the familiar words:"Remember, what the doctor told you?" This profession is so highly regarded and rewarded by our society, yet so little is known about the "inside information" on how medicine is actually practiced. Yes, anyone knows what doctors' office look like, what hospitals look like and how x-rays are done. But very few know how medical practice actually works. They do not understand what actually goes through the minds of the doctors and nurses when they are evaluating a patient. They do not understand how doctors eventually arrive at the diagnosis and treatment plans that they make every day. They do not understand how much doctors can rely on the blood tests and x-rays and how much they cannot. They do not understand how much influence the age, gender, occupation, personal habits and family background of a patient can have on the diagnosis the doctor considers.

From the explanation so far, it appears as if there are two very different worlds of medicine that do not coincide with each other. One seen from the eyes of a doctor, and one seen from the eyes of everyone else. This book is an attempt to show a regular person the world of medicine as seen from the eyes of the doctor. Books of this nature are very difficult to find for a few reasons. First of all, most doctors have already forgotten how they felt (or how everyone else feels) about medical profession before they went into it. Second, they find it a waste of time trying to explain the reason behind the medical decision. They feel that, without the scientific medical knowledge, any detailed explanation would be incomprehensible and therefore useless. Thirdly, by revealing the doubts, uncertainties and imperfections of the medical science, they fear losing the confidence of their patients. This is why all medical advice tend to be in an authoritative and overly factual tone with conscious skipping of the uncertainties and doubts. Most of the medical books that are written for the general readers so far only offer some form of medical advice or opinion.

The few books that attempt to give the readers a doctor's view of medicine are mostly personal stories rather than factual information.

This book is different in that it does not give you any medical advice but tells you how modern clinical medicine works. It explains to you in a simple factual manner how doctors process the information obtained from your blood tests and what goes through the doctors' mind when they ask you a particular question. It tells you what the doctor is listening for when he puts the stethoscope in your chest. It gives you interesting facts about what doctors learn in medical school and what they learn outside the medical school. It tells you how medical students and doctors at different stages of their training interact with each other and how that might influence your hospital experience. It explains to you about why they do screening tests for certain diseases and not for others. It explains to you what it means when the media reports the findings of a new drug research. In summary, it gives you the little secrets that are taken for granted in the medical profession but would be very surprising and exciting to the outsiders.

I, myself, had all these doubts before I decided to write this book. I happened to remember and cherish my memory and my feeling towards medical profession before I went into it. But, I too was immersed in the technical details of the medical world during my medical school and during my clinical training. When I started my medical practice, I tried to be more passionate and looked directly into the patient's eyes and started seeing the human being in front of me. I tried to find out not only about how her organs are working, but also about how she is feeling about seeing the doctor and being in the hospital. Slowly, this refreshed my memory, I started to remember how I felt about medicine and doctors before I became one of them. After I realized there are two different worlds of medicine, I attempted to show the doctor's world of medicine to the patients, but again held myself back as I had doubts that they would understand it. I, too, had doubts that these revelations would make me less authoritative.

Subsequently, I realized that, the hospital or the doctor's office was not the best place to explain these secrets of the medical world to the people of non-medical background. I then started to answer questions of friends and family over dinner conversations and discovered how interested and excited people were to hear about these "little secrets" of the medical world. I realized that after knowing these secrets, they did not have any doubts or any less respect for their doctors. Instead, they were able to better understand why their doctors behave the way they do. After knowing about the imperfections and limitations of modern medicine, they had more respect for their doctors knowing how many things the doctor has to consider before making a particular decision. These experiences aroused a very strong desire in me, a desire to build a bridge — a bridge between the two very different worlds of medicines.

I strongly feel that there is a need for this bridge between these two different worlds of medicine and I am confident that this bridge can be built and maintained. I invite you, the intelligent reader, to cross this bridge with me. You are welcome to this world which has been kept as a secret from you — a world of medicine as seen from the eye of the doctor. You can now explore the methods, weakness, strength, excitement, joys and sorrows of modern medicine.

Chapter 2: How does the doctor find out what is wrong with you?

Well, basically, you tell him.

That is right. Even with the availability of sophisticated blood tests , highly advanced imaging with CT scan, MRI and nuclear scans, very advanced medical equipment and endoscopic procedures, the most important piece of information the doctor needs to make a diagnosis is what you tell him. This part of your medical evaluation is called the "history taking" and this is the single most important piece of information that leads to the correct diagnosis. This part of the medical evaluation also demands a high degree of skill and patience on the part of the doctor as well as the patient.

The patient is in pain. She is in agony. She wants to be treated fast. She wants to get that x-ray done right away. She wants to get that antibiotic started right away. She is in no mood to go over what happened and what she was doing when the pain started. But the doctor has to know everything, he just needs all the answers. He keeps asking all these seemingly stupid questions. He wants to know how many cigarettes the patient smoked. He even wants to know what meal the patient had and what time the last meal was. He also wants to know if the patient had any beer or wine with the meal. He does not stop at that. He even wants to know how many beers did she have with the meal. He is also asking if the patient has lost any weight recently. The patient is getting impatient. She is tired of answering all these questions. She wonders why she is being interrogated instead of being helped.

This is a very common scenario in an emergency department or at a hospital bed. The patient can get very frustrated and angry with all these questions. Not only the patient, it can also be very frustrating for the inexperienced clinician or a student doctor, and sometimes even to an experienced doctor. There are certain methods and certain techniques of this process called history taking.

Although most of my patients continue to answer my questions as I keep asking them, I can see the surprise, agony, anxiety and sometimes frustration in their eyes as to why they have to answer all these details. I almost wish at one of those times that they would stop me and ask me why I wanted to know all the details. I always wish I could take some time to explain why I needed to ask them so many details about their personal life as a part of the medical evaluation. But then I realize that when someone is sick and suffering, that is not the best time to explain about the reasoning and goals of this process called "comprehensive history taking". I will try to explain it here to all of you when you have the curiosity and time to read my book.

Symptoms of a disease and their relation to the disease that causes the particular symptom seem very straight forward. We hear about them all the time. We have commercials from the pharmaceutical companies on TV explaining what symptoms are caused by what disease and they want you to ask your doctor about a particular medicine. You also have programs on TV and radio stations where you listen to health care professionals talk about the symptoms to look for when you are worried about a particular disease. You hear about a certain disease and it's symptoms during public information campaign organized by different groups. Interestingly, whenever any celebrity or public figure is diagnosed with any disease or condition, you keep hearing about that disease in details on the media for weeks or sometimes for months. The common theme in all these sources of information tends to be the same. They have one disease, then they have 3 or 4 symptoms, the name of the medicine to treat the disease, or the name of the surgical procedure to correct that condition. Subsequently, these medical terms become household names.

When you hear about different diseases, different

symptoms and different treatments over some period of time, your brain starts to process the information in a particular manner and you tend to form a pattern about diseases and symptoms. It will then seem to you that there are a set of symptoms a patient can have and there are a set of diseases that are represented by one or more of the symptoms. It would then seem logical that you should make a simple table with 2 columns and put the names of the diseases on the left side and the names of the symptoms on the other side and match them. If you can correctly match the set of the symptoms with a particular disease, you have the knowledge to be able to suggest the diagnosis based on the symptoms the patient is having. In fact, this is the most common perception of disease and diagnosis that is present not only in the general

> The general thinking is that there is a set of symptoms a patient can have and there is a set of diseases that are represented by one or more of these symptoms. If this were true, we could develop a computerized algorithm that could match the symptoms to the disease and make the diagnosis. This could potentially replace doctors with computers and bring down the health care costs significantly.

population but also in the majority of para-medical and other entry level health profession.

If we extend these concepts further it seems logical that someone should program the above mentioned facts into a computer software. If you create a computer algorithm where you could match the symptoms to the diseases, you could be solving a lot of problems. For example, you could enter the symptoms you are having into the system and it could match your symptoms to a particular disease and suggest a diagnosis. Then you could also have a second algorithm where the computer could match the recently diagnosed disease with the best available treatment option and now you have a treatment plan. Maybe, this is exactly what we need to do to bring down the cost of medicine: replace doctors with computers!

Wait a minute! Do not be over exited yet. This is not a new concept. And, in fact, such programs already exist. There are many websites where you can get these results quickly. Now, you may be wondering: “Then, what's the catch? Why don’t we all use these programs instead of waiting in long lines to see the doctor?”

The concept of the “set of symptoms” and “set of diseases” is a little more complex than that. In fact, physicians do not even think of medicine as sets of symptoms and diseases. Each symptom is only a small clue to what particular part of the body organ system might have been affected by the disease process. Then the doctor has to think about which part of the organ could have been involved. Then the next question would be what kind of process could have affected that particular part of that organ. Note that, at this point, I am talking about “process”. The process could be a shortage of blood supply, a swelling, an injury, an abnormal growth or any other type of bodily function that can go wrong with the organ. It is only in the latter part of the decision making process that the doctors think about what disease could have affected that particular part of that organ to cause that particular process which can result in the presenting symptom.

Somewhat confused?

Let me try to explain this with an example. Some of you may have heard about the disease pneumonia. If not, it is a type of infection of the lungs. You may have also heard about the two common symptoms of pneumonia — cough and fever. Now let us use the computer algorithm model of medicine first. It is very simple. You just enter the two symptoms, and let the computer do the matching. Then you are done. You get your answer. You “have” pneumonia. That’s it. That is your disease. You have diagnosed your disease. Now let's explore the same problem from the doctor's point of view.

The patient is having cough. Now the doctor has to first figure out which organ could have been affected. At first, it seems like a silly question. You have a cough. It is obviously your lungs, isn't it? Isn't that where you cough from? In reality, it is not that simple. In fact, cough could be related to nose, throat, lungs, food pipe or even stomach. That is why he needs to know more details about the cough. First, he needs to know how it started. If it started with sneezing and runny nose, it could be related to the nose. Sometimes when you get a runny nose, you may have some of the drainage from the runny nose drip back into your throat and that could be the reason for the cough. After a series of detailed questions, he is now able to make an assumption that this particular cough in this patient is coming from the lungs(I have used the plural form "lungs" as you have two lungs). Now he has to find out which part of the lungs could it be coming from.

Here, when I talk about part, it does not necessarily mean which side which corner or how deep. It also means which component of the lungs. The lungs seem like two big organs from the outside, but they have many components. They have the large air pipe which is called trachea. It is like the stem or the bottom large part of a tree. The trachea or the main pipe then divides into two branches and go into each lung. These two big branches are called bronchus. After they go inside the lungs, they further divide into other smaller branches. These small branches of the air pipe are called bronchioles. They subsequently form a small air sac. Each air sac is called alveolus. Now, besides these air pipes and air sacs, the lungs also have other components. They have the blood vessels that also divide into different components. Then they also have connecting tissue that holds the different blood vessels, air tubes and air sacs together. Then they also have a thin plastic like membrane that covers the whole lungs.

Now, to the doctor, the "lung cough" could be coming from any of these components of the lungs. That is why he has to know very specific details about the cough. He has to know if it is a hoarse barking type cough or a dry hacking type cough. Is it a wet cough that ends up with expectoration of green foul smelling sputum or is it a dry cough with a production of small white colored sputum? Is it a continuous cough that happens throughout the day or is it an intermittent cough that happens mostly when the patient tries to speak? Does it hurt when the patient coughs? If it hurts, which side of the chest hurts when coughing? These are some of the questions the doctor needs to ask in order to find out which component of the lungs the cough is originating from.

After he has an idea of which component of the lungs the cough is coming from, he would like to know what kind of process could be going on in there. Is it a problem of decreased blood supply caused by a blood clot in that particular part of the lungs? Is it a swelling in that area of the lungs? Is it an infection? Could there be a small tumor or cancer in that part of the lungs? Could the patient have inhaled any harmful chemical substance that has caused some injury to the particular component of the lungs? These are only a few examples of processes that can go wrong in the lungs all of which could result in the symptom cough.

To explore these possibilities, the doctor has to ask a few more questions. He needs to know if the patient had any problems with blood clots in the past. He needs to know if the patient has used any birth control pills as that is one of the risk factors for increased blood clots. He needs to know if anyone in the patient's family had blood clots. He needs to know if the patient had ever suffered from asthma which is caused by swelling of the small air pipes of the lungs. He needs to know if the patient smoked cigarettes. He also needs to know how many cigarettes a day did the patient smoke and also needs to know how many years she smoked for. He needs to know what kind of work the patient does to see if the patient could have been exposed to any type of chemical substance. He needs to know if the patient works in a dusty place. He needs to know if the patient works at a place with lots of pollen in the air. He needs to know if the patient lives in a crowded dormitory where it is easy to catch an infection. He needs to know about the patient's sexual practices to see if the patient could have a higher risk of catching a sexually transmitted disease that can settle down in a particular component of the lungs.

I wish I could explain why I am asking each question before I ask it. But that is not practically possible during the actual patient interview because of the time it would take and because of the anxiety it might provoke. After all, the patient's main desire is to finish all that question/answer session and to get the treatment as soon as possible to get better.

Now let us explore a simple doctor patient encounter systematically and find out how and what types of questions the doctor will ask. When someone presents to the emergency department with a complaint of chest pain, that patient is very anxious to know what could be the reason for her pain. The patient is very eager to be "seen" by the doctor. She is anxious to know what the doctor would find out after listening to her heart with the stethoscope. She is already ready to take those deep breaths for the lung exam. To the patient the most awaited reassurance would be if the doctor tells the patient that the heart sounds are normal or the lungs sound clear. The patient would be very happy and relieved to hear those physical findings from the doctor. That is an important piece of information. But to the doctor, that is only a small part of the picture. In fact only a very small number of patients with an acute heart attack have an abnormal finding on the heart or the lung exam. Therefore, the doctor evaluating the patient with a chest pain is not at all reassured by the normal heart and lung exam.

Then, you must be wondering how the doctor decides which patients to reassure and send home and which patients to keep for further evaluation of a possible heart attack. Your first instinct would be to say: "Do some tests and find out." If you have been with me so far, you probably guessed that the answer is wrong. Then, what is the most important piece of information the doctor considers in making this decision? You guessed it right — it is what the patient tells the doctor. And the best way of getting this important information is to encourage the patient to come forward with the information voluntarily so as to avoid asking yes or no questions. The doctor starts asking open ended general questions first.

For example, he might ask, "What were you doing when the pain started?" or "How did it start?" or "Tell me what made you decide to come to the hospital today?"

With these questions, the doctor hopes to get unbiased and complete information surrounding the event. On the other hand if he had asked a more specific,"Were you doing heavy physical exercise when the pain started?", the patient's response could have been less specific. Heavy physical exercise may signify different things to different patients. It is, therefore, critical to get an accurate and actual description of what they were doing instead of generalized answers.

But this question can sometimes get different unintended response. When asked,"What were you doing when the pain started?", the patient might respond: "Why? nothing." With that answer, patient goes into a defensive mode as she thinks that the question implies that the patient is responsible for bringing the pain to herself by doing something.

The most helpful answer would be a simple description of events before the pain started. For example, "I was sitting on the couch watching TV and suddenly noticed some kind of burning pain in the chest/neck area." or "I went out to shovel the snow and after I shoveled for 10 minutes, I felt very tired and dizzy and started having this heaviness in my chest." These are the types of answers that actually help the doctor a lot to make these types of complex decisions.

The next most important question the doctor will ask is how exactly did the patient feel. This conversation can also turn awkward if the patient second guesses the doctor's intention. For example if someone had a bad chest pain and went to the ER and the doctor asks,"What did the pain feel like?" the patient can sometimes be startled with the question. She might think, "What does he think it feels like to have pain?" The most unhelpful answer would be,"Of coarse, I felt very bad when I had the pain." The most helpful answer would be, "It felt like an elephant was sitting on my chest." or "It felt like something was burning and churning inside my chest." The other way to get this information is to ask the patient: "What type of pain you had?" This question has less of a chance to offend anyone but is also slightly inferior in its ability to be able to bring forward the most helpful information. The problem with this question is that patients do not always know how many types of pains are out there and often do not recognize and describe the type of pain. They might ask: "What do you mean by what type of pain? It was just pain — really bad pain." Then the next step for the doctor would be to give the patient a multiple choice question by asking, "Was it a sharp cutting type pain or dull burning ache or twisty cramp-like pain or heavy pressure type pain?" If the doctor has to go all the way to this step to be able to get a description of the pain, then the information obtained would be less helpful. Giving a closed ended multiple choice question at this point severely limits the full descriptive narrative of the pain which is really important for the doctor. Also different patients perceive pain differently. Some may perceive a tightness as a pressure and some may perceive it as squeezing. After the doctor has obtained the full description of the pain and a complete description of the surrounding events when the pain started, he has already obtained the most important first step in making the diagnosis.

Once the doctor is able to obtain the detailed information about the "onset" or circumstances surrounding the start of the symptoms and the quality or detailed description of the subjective feeling associated with the pain, he is already starting to make a mental picture of what organ systems could have been involved. He then starts making plans about what further specific questions to ask and what to focus on the physical exam. From now on his questions are less awkward and more specific and less difficult to answer.

The next thing he would want to know is the severity of the pain. That is, it is only now that he wants to know how bad the pain is. The patient is usually very forthcoming to answer that question.

"When 0 is no pain at all and 10 is the worst pain you can ever imagine, what rating would you give your pain?"

This is an easy enough question but is a very important one. It not only helps in pointing towards the right diagnosis but also helps to track response to the treatment. For example, if it was rated at 8 before the treatment and it is now a 4, it means that the treatment did have some effect on the patient's symptoms.

Next thing the doctor needs to know is the "radiation" of the pain. It simply means where the pain goes from its original place of occurrence. This information is easy to obtain by asking a simple question, "Does your pain stay there or does it move to somewhere else?" This helps the doctor to think about which organs might be involved and which nerve pathway the pain might have traveled.

This information cannot be simply obtained by listening to your chest with a stethoscope. Only your body, your mind and your nerves have all the inside information to your internal organ system and the maximum amount of information can only be obtained by asking questions directly to you. Your body has a way of telling you about the disease process by making you feel pain and discomfort in a certain way and the doctor tries to interpret these messages by asking you detailed question. If you are able describe things in a very elaborate way, you are giving the doctor a very important tool for the diagnosis. If you can give the doctor a detailed description of the exact onset, location, quality and radiation of the pain, you are directly conveying the information that your diseased organs are trying to tell you.

The interview is not over yet. The doctor still has to know a few more things about your pain before moving on to other general health questions. The next information to be obtained is about the exacerbating factors. A simple question ,"What seems to make your pain worse?" is usually sufficient to obtain this information. This step, in combination with the ameliorating factors, helps the doctor make certain inferences about what kind of disease process the organ system might be having.

One more thing the doctor has to ask about the pain is "associated symptoms". Different approaches are taken to get this information. A very open ended question will be asked first such as, "Have you had any other symptoms besides the pain itself?" or "Was the pain associated with any other symptoms or discomfort?" After the first open ended approach, a next more direct closed ended questions will follow. "Did you get dizzy when you had the pain?" "Were you having trouble breathing when you had the pain?" The combined information obtained from all these questions gives the doctor a very clear direction as to which diseases and organ systems to pursue for further testing. Without this information, doing tests blindly is like "looking for a needle in a haystack." When you know which exact area to explore, it will be easier to find what you need. Otherwise, there are hundreds of thousands of different medical tests that are done to diagnose thousands of diseases. If you did all these tests in a patient, chances are that you will find some abnormal finding in some patients but you will not be able to tell whether the abnormal finding is significant or not. I will be discussing medical tests and their significance in a whole different chapter (chapter 4).

Chapter 3: Why does the doctor always ask me so many irrelevant questions?

After reading the previous chapter, you probably know why the details of the cough and chest pain are important and you also probably figured out how the doctor might ask questions in order to get these answers. But the part of the medical history taking (part of doctor's questions) that might make you uncomfortable and anxious is not over yet.

The first part of this extended information gathering is called "Past Medical History (PMH)". The one important thing to remember about this part is that it is an integral part of the medical history that is asked during every medical encounter. It does not matter if you are in for just a regular visit or presenting to ER with chest pain, the doctor needs to know what kind of medical problems you had in the past . Without this information, the doctor will have a hard time putting together your symptoms in the right context. The Past Medical History is like a background information or a road map that will help put your current problem in the right context and help connect the dots to look at the bigger picture.

Let's assume we have two different patients who are identical except for their Past Medical History. The first one had 3 surgeries in his abdomen over a course of many years but the second one had not had any surgery in the past. Now, let us go back to the previous chapter and think about the things that could be asked in the first part of the interview. After a detailed history, let us say both patients had the pain started the same way, had the same type of pain, had the same intensity of pain. Both of them had the pain worsened by similar things and improved with similar measures. Both these patients had nausea and vomiting associated with the pain. When the doctor starts to ask questions about Past Medical History, he discovers about the surgeries that one of the two patients had. After getting this information, his approach to these two patients will differ completely.

There are certain things that happen more often in patients who had prior abdominal surgery than in patients without any history of surgery. The doctor may decide to do some additional tests in the patient with prior surgeries. He may also decide to keep that patient in the hospital overnight to watch him more closely but may send the other patient home with some pain medicines. In this way, past medical problems provide a context to evaluate patient's current symptoms. In this case, two patients with the exact same symptoms will receive completely different treatments because of the difference in their Past Medical History.

After the Past Medical History, questions will be directed towards any allergies to any medications or any food products. The reason for this question is fairly obvious and easy to understand. They want to know about allergies to avoid using that medication in that particular patient. Sometimes, the doctor wants to know what exactly happened when you had the allergic reaction. It is important in certain cases where the doctor still plans to use certain life saving medication despite the allergy. Sometimes that becomes necessary where the alternative medicine is less effective. If the allergy to the medication was a minor reaction or just an upset stomach, he may still consider to use it if absolutely needed.

The next question would be about medications that the patient is taking. When telling your doctor about your medications, it is important to include over the counter medications and herbal products or nutritional supplements too. Most of the over the counter medications are active "pharmacological chemicals" or drugs that alter body functions. They can cause serious side effects or even organ damage or death if taken improperly or in the wrong dose. Some of them also interact with other prescription medications and can cause serious illness by either greatly enhancing the effects of the prescription drug or by neutralizing its effect. Even herbal products or nutritional supplements may have active chemicals that can cause similar effects. It is therefore very important to give a detailed and complete list of all the medications you are taking. When you are sick enough to visit an emergency department, you should consider taking all your pill bottles with you. If you actually take the pill bottles instead of the list of your medication, it can make things easier for the doctors and the nurses. The pill bottle will have more information than just the drug name and dosing. With the pill bottle, you will be able to tell when that particular pill was prescribed, when the last refill was given and what exact strength pill was used. Actual pill bottle will

> Questions about past medical problems give the doctor the background information needed to evaluate current symptoms. Without properly understanding patient's social, family and job situation, it is difficult to put the current symptoms in the right context.

also make it harder to mistake one drug for another because of “sound alike” or “look alike” medications.

The reason behind asking a complete medication list is also fairly easy to comprehend and patients normally do not have many questions about it. Another advantage of having a complete list of medication is that it can alert your doctor about your chronic medical problems that you might have missed to mention in the Past Medical History. When confronted with a medication on the list that does not match your Past Medical History, the doctor might simply ask you: “Do you know what was the reason for your doctor to give you this particular pill?” That might refresh your memory and you might start talking about one of your medical conditions that you forgot to mention.

With the next few questions, things can sometimes get a

little awkward. Now it is time for "personal and social" questions. Most of the times, patients feel uneasy with these questions as they fail to understand why these questions carry any significance at all. At other times, they may feel like they are being judged by the doctor with these questions.

Why does the doctor need to know what kind of job you do? Why does the doctor need to know what kind of place you live in? Why does the doctor need to know how many people are there in your family?

By this time, you have learned the importance of the subjective symptoms reported by the patient in determining the correct diagnosis and help guide the doctor to order the right tests and procedures. The whole idea behind the extended interview is to place everything in context. You can probably understand that what people do for a living has usually some effect on how they feel pain or pressure For example, for a person used to doing manual labor that requires heavy lifting or pushing, occasional muscle pain here and there may be perceived as "normal". An executive who sits on his desk all day may be very concerned by any pain on her shoulder or low back. Also, certain diseases and conditions are related to certain occupations. For example "carpel tunnel syndrome" almost exclusively happens in people whose job involves a lot of typing or writing. Certain animal related diseases occur in people whose occupation requires close contact to those animals. Health care workers such as doctors and nurses are at risk of developing infection with more resistant organisms as their occupation involves daily close contact with multiple types of worms and bugs.

If a patient lives alone, she might be somewhat reluctant to report certain symptoms like weakness or lethargy. If that person had been living with several family members, someone would have noticed these changes. Certain symptoms can only be seen and reported by others. For example if a patient had seizures, she would be unconscious during the episode and only others would be able to describe what the patient did during the seizure.

This is how a person's lifestyle, occupation and family gives us the background information needed to interpret the symptoms in a unique way. By our discussion so far, it is clear that most of the information needed to accurately make a diagnosis is actually the kind of information that is very subjective and depends more on knowing the whole person in front of the doctor rather than just relying on a quick physical exam. Without properly understanding your social background and your occupation, it is difficult to evaluate your symptoms in the right context.

Medical diagnosis making is in some way similar to a detective work. These days, even detectives rely on DNA testing. Without a proper story that fits the person's profile and a possible theory of what could have happened, the DNA test in itself has very limited role for the detective. In the same way, without having a background knowledge about a patient's Past Medical History and current social situation, it will be very difficult to put the significance of medical tests in the right context.

The next few questions will be about your personal habits and addictions. This part can be very uncomfortable to some patients. You are really concerned about the cough you are having for the last few weeks and finally find a time to visit your doctor and he asks: "Do you smoke cigarettes?"

At that time you may feel uneasy and start to think ,"So, he thinks my cough is from my smoking" or "He wants to blame everything on my smoking."

Or, if you never smoked or hated cigarettes all your life, you might think: "What makes him think that I would smoke cigarettes?"

This way the patient may feel like she is being judged by the doctor when she hears these words. Questions about tobacco, alcohol and illicit drugs are parts of this very important component of the medical interview. Actually, doctors ask these questions to all patients precisely because they do not want to be judgmental. They do not pick and choose which patient needs to be questioned about alcohol and drugs and which ones do not.

Tobacco abuse or cigarette smoking affects every organ system in the body and the chemical in tobacco "nicotine" is a very active pharmacological (like medicines) chemical and has very significant effects on the human body and its different organ systems including blood, heart, brain and lungs to name a few. It is therefore very important to know if that person has ever been exposed to this substance. It not only helps to assess overall risks for different health problems but also helps to make the correct diagnosis. Certain medical problems almost exclusively happen in smokers. One example is a disease called Chronic Obstructive Pulmonary Disease or COPD. It is very rare to have COPD in non-smokers. In patients presenting with a cough and breathing problem that has been going for a long time, the kind of tests the doctor orders depends on whether the patient smokes cigarettes or not. It is therefore very important to find out if the patient smokes.

It is also important to find out how many packs of cigarettes the patient smokes and how many years has she smoked for. It is also important to know about past smoking even though the patient quit smoking many years ago. Most of the changes in your body from smoking start getting better after you quit smoking. The earlier you quit, the less will be the effects remaining in your body. But unfortunately, it does not go back to normal even after many years. It is, therefore, important to know about any remote history of cigarette smoking in addition to recent history. The doctors use a term "pack-year" to describe the total sum of cigarettes that a person has smoked throughout her life. If the patient smoked about 1 pack of cigarettes a day and has been smoking for 30 year, then the "pack-year" sum of total smoking is obtained by multiplying the total number of years of smoking by average "pack of cigarettes smoked per day. A "pack" is assumed to be 20 cigarettes. This number gives the doctor the rough estimate of risk of certain diseases in smokers.

Knowledge about patient's smoking also helps to plan a

patient's hospital coarse after an elective surgery or other unrelated problems. For example, if someone who smokes cigarettes is in the hospital for an elective knee replacement surgery, that person will need to be monitored more carefully after the surgery as she might develop pneumonia or lung infection more easily than other patients with similar problems but no history of cigarette smoking.

Similarly, when questioning about alcohol use, it is also very important to know how many drinks the patient has in a day or in a week and how many years has she been using alcohol. It is specially important with questions about alcohol to include minute details as small amount of alcohol is socially acceptable and even might have some beneficial effects to the body. Knowledge about the type, amount, frequency and previous alcohol related social and legal problems help the doctor in making decision about patient's diagnosis, treatment and monitoring. It is equally true whether the patient's symptoms are related to alcohol or not.

Let us again consider the example of the patient who came to the hospital for a knee surgery. Although the reason she is in the hospital is completely unrelated to alcohol use, history of alcohol use is very helpful in monitoring her health after the surgery. If she was a habitual heavy drinker, she is at a very high risk of developing certain symptoms that would need specialized treatment. If things get really bad, she could even have life threatening seizure from the alcohol withdrawal. At the same time, let me mention one interesting fact about knee pain and alcohol use. Try to think of a situation when alcohol use could directly cause knee pain. Yes, that is right. Alcohol use can cause falls and accidents and that can cause knee pain. This one is obvious and easy to understand. But there is another condition called "gout" which you might have heard about. Patients with prior history of this problem are at high risk of developing knee pain or gout pain whenever they are dehydrated. In addition to causing dehydration, alcohol can actually directly increase the chances of having a "gout attack" and can cause knee pain. After all, knee pain does not seem to be totally unrelated to alcohol use, does it?

After the questions about alcohol, the next question is usually about illicit drug use. After explaining the medical importance of tobacco and alcohol , it might be easier to explain the logic behind asking questions about any other drug use. It may not be difficult to understand that all street drugs are active chemicals that alter bodily function in a very significant way. But unlike tobacco or alcohol, street drugs are not socially acceptable and are illegal. For this reason, people who actually use street drugs are very confrontational about the question and want to lie about it unless they are convinced by the doctor about the importance of that information. On the other hand, people who do not use drugs feel very strange to be asked about street drugs. They will start thinking about why the doctor could have asked such a question and wonder what is it about them that could make the doctor suspect drug use. But that is the exact reason why doctors ask it to everyone and not pick and choose anyone based on their appearance or behavior to ask these questions.

The last component of the extended medical history is called the "review of systems". So far, I have been telling you that the doctor mostly tries to get full and detailed information about the symptoms to get the big picture. But now, this last part is a little different. This will be a last check list that will mostly ask yes/no questions and expect a short answer. For this part, the doctor will ask you a set of seemingly unrelated questions about all your organ systems that are not related to your main problem. For example if you went to the hospital with abdominal pain, you will first be asked about the details of your abdominal pain and then you will be asked all about your past medical problems, your medications, your social situation and your family situation. Finally, you will be asked if you have any headaches, any fever, any chest pain, any shortness of breath etc. This step seems like a final checklist of unrelated problems and it is exactly that. It is a review of all body symptoms to make sure that there was no symptom that the patient forgot to talk about or did not consider important enough to mention.

The interview has been going on for some time now and the patient is anxious to be actually "examined" by the doctor. But now you understand that by this time the doctor has obtained the most important information to make the diagnosis. Details about the "medical exam" also called physical exam will be discussed in a separate chapter.

Chapter 4: My test was normal. I do not have the disease, do I?

Well, not that simple.

Medical decision making is a very complex process. Some of you may be surprised to know that modern medicine, no matter how advanced it is, is not a complete science in the absolute sense of the word. The methods of modern medicine are quite different from the way science and technology works in other fields. A rocket scientist relies upon knowledge of physics to calculate the velocity required to propel a rocket into the outer space from the earth. He relies upon the knowledge of chemistry to calculate the amount of fuel required to generate the energy for the chemical reaction to get the rocket propelled with the exact velocity he devises. He calculates the direction of the rocket by the physical properties of its structure, its density, its geometry and three dimensional structures. His methods are strictly scientific and calculated by complex but factual knowledge. They can and do predict things with high degree of scientific accuracy.

> We hear about miraculous sounding new medical breakthroughs every month on TV. Most people have heard about artificial hearts and artificial kidneys. When we hear see and read about these types of advancement in the medical field, it is not surprising that most people think of modern medicine as an advanced science.

We hear, read and see about advancement in medical field everyday. We watch about medical breakthroughs every month on TV. Some of us may have heard about the human genome project which was completed successfully. It was a huge project performed by medical scientists all over the world. They were able to crack all the codes in the human DNA. Most people have heard about artificial hearts, artificial kidneys.

When we are surrounded and bombarded by so much information about advancement in modern medicine, we start to believe that modern medicine is an advanced science just like rocket science or computer technology. One tends to believe that doctors and hospitals have the ability to diagnose and treat human diseases with 100% accuracy and scientific certainty.

In the real world, those are far from 100% accurate. In fact, no test in medicine is 100% accurate, no matter how advanced state of the art technology has been used to do that test.

With this being said, let us explore the science and technology used in medical diagnostics. Knowledge of general chemistry as well as organic chemistry applied to medical diagnostics is very advanced. A simple blood test can accurately analyze the chemical constituents of our blood. It can accurately determine the amount of sodium, potassium or even the amount of alcohol or other toxins in the blood. It can count the different type of cells that are floating in the liquid part of the blood called serum. It can also accurately determine the oxygen and nutrients and different proteins in the blood. With some advanced tests, it can also determine the different types of special proteins that are made by our body to perform special tasks. Some of these special proteins are called enzymes. They perform a specific task during the production of a specific active product that can carry out a unique biological function to maintain the vital function of our body. Thousands of such enzymes have been discovered and extensively studied and very accurate tests exist to both qualitatively and quantitatively detect these proteins in the body.

Scientific knowledge of physics applied in medical diagnostics is equally advanced, amazing and fascinating. We all have seen x-ray films that are shadow pictures of internal organs. Well, x-rays have evolved quite a bit in the last 20 years. With advanced computerized CAT scan machines, it is possible now to take pictures of every internal organ with a resolution of less than a few millimeters. What that means is that you can see all the internal organs up to a detail of a few millimeters on a computer screen just like you can use Google earth to view details of landscape, roads and houses and even cars in your own neighborhood. With the use of radioactive isotopes it is even possible to trace the activity of certain cells and certain enzymes in the body. Advanced Magnetic Resonance Imaging (MRI) machines are able to detect even a small deposit of calcium inside a blood vessel or a very small area of plaque in the brain. And there are nuclear medicine scanners that can even detect small increase in blood flow or small inflammation inside the cells of your bone.

To this point you may be wondering why, even with such modern and advanced technology, is medical science not a real science and why is it not as accurate as rocket science. Well, to answer this question, we will have to explore a whole new aspect of medicine — the "human" factor in medicine.

> With the advanced technology used in the medical field, we almost tend to forget that the objective of modern medicine is to treat humans. This "human factor" is the main reason that modern medicine is not an exact science.

All medical students are taught that medicine is a combination of art and science. The scientific part of medicine is obvious and easy to understand. But medicine as an art? In this technologically advanced world , it may come as a surprise to you. It may be easier to understand it if we go back to the basics of medical science. No matter how advanced the science and technology used, the subjects of medical practice are living human beings just like you and me. If you look around you in your office, you see people, all of them look different. Each person has his/her own personality.

Let's say, you are at a friend's house, on a Saturday afternoon enjoying some beer and watching football. The game is on and your team is leading. All your friends are supporting the same team and suddenly the other team makes a strike. Everyone is sad and says or does something in response. But if you observe carefully, you will notice that everyone reacts to the same situation differently or at least the expression of the same feeling is quite different in different individuals. Some may frown their eyebrows and hit the couch with the right hand. Some may sit back and scream. Some may stand up and make a fist. No two individuals express the same emotion in an identical way.

After the game is over, your friends decide to have a barbeque and some beer. You will notice that the beer has slightly different effect on every one. Some get drowsy and sleepy, others get more alert and some start smiling in a funny way.

The above examples show that different human beings react differently to same emotions and also behave differently under the influence of the same substance. At a glance, all humans are similar but if you explore the details, each human being is a like a unique work of art. This is where the art of medicine comes from. This is where the similarity between a doctor and a car repair technician ends. A car mechanic has to know the make, model and trim of a vehicle and he will know the exact details about what type of engine and what parts are in it. For doctors, every patient is a unique human being and no two human beings are identical in any aspect. This uniqueness is more than just in their external appearances. This is in every organ system and in the biochemical composition of every bodily fluid. Every liver is different. Every kidney is different. The composition of everyone's blood is different. The way each person's immune system handles infection is different. Every brain is different and the amount and type of chemical messenger in every human brain is different. It is this difference that gives all of us a unique identity.

One may wonder and ask how is it possible to engineer humans in a way that each of us is unique yet functional human being. If you think about the auto industry, just imagine how much work would it require to create every single car that is fundamentally different from every other car not only in the body and color, but also in the engine and transmission.

The secret of this variability actually lies in our secret organs. Yes, sexual reproduction is the only mechanism created by mother nature to ensure that each of her offspring is uniquely different and has its own personality. How is that possible? The answer lies in our genes and DNA. Everyone must have heard these two words as they are used everywhere from Hollywood science fiction movies to TV crime shows and day-time reality TV shows. Actually, genes are the biological units that we inherit from our parents. DNA is the basic organic structure that genes are made up of. In essence our genes have programs that determine our body composition including not only our hair color, eye shape but also our blood type, our heart, our kidneys and even our brains. Genes exist in pairs. We inherit one gene from each parent and one pair of gene determines one particular trait of our body. The fate of our hair color or eye shape is decided by the gene pairing at the time we are fertilized.

The mechanism by which mother nature ensures that everyone is different occurs at the time when our sperms and eggs are made. When sperms are made, the DNA in the cells that eventually become sperms break into thousands of pieces and then they re-arrange themselves just like shuffling a deck of cards. This shuffling is the basic step how mother nature gambles with our future just to make sure everyone gets a different fate in his/her life. This shuffling takes place both while making eggs and sperms. Millions of sperms are made everyday and each one of them has had the shuffling done before it is ready. This way every single sperm has a unique set of genes. Only one of the luckiest single sperm will meet its other half (the egg) and will get a new life. This is the life we all know. All the others that do not meet their love of life will die away within 72 hours.

Interesting story, but what does this have to do with my test result? Well, I am getting there. To this point, we have learned how each individual is different. Just like expression of happiness, anger and effects of alcohol are different in different individuals, the presentation of a particular disease is also slightly different in different individuals.

Even members of a single family that catch common cold with the same virus do not have the exact same symptoms. Let's pick up on one symptom everyone knows. People get sneezing when they catch a cold. Does everyone have the same amount of sneezing when they catch a cold? No. In fact some of them may not sneeze at all and still have other symptoms of common cold such as stuffy nose, headache and mild fever. Does everyone who have sneezing has a common cold? No. You occasionally sneeze when you get some pungent odor or dust or pollen in your house. We explored this simple question "Sneezing or no sneezing?" in diagnosing common cold. The same principle applies to all human disease processes no matter how complex they are. In the above example the question "Do you have sneezing?" can be regarded as a medical test. The answer to the question "yes" or "no" can be regarded as the result of the medical diagnostic testing. In this case, if the test is positive do you have the disease? Not always. If the test is negative, are you free from disease? Not always.

In practice, the setting or the situation which you have before the test determines the significance of the test result. If you see a person who seems to have common cold as she has runny nose with mild fever and you ask her,"Do you have sneezing too?" and she says,"Yes", you will be more certain that she does have a common cold. If it is someone who just came out of a flower shop and has sneezing, you do not think that she has a cold even though her answer to the above question would be affirmative. In medical terms, this quality is called the "Pretest Probability" and is as important as the result of the test itself. There are thousands of different blood tests, urine tests as well as tests of other different types of fluids that are present in the different organs of the body. All these tests measure different chemicals and different cells that are present in these fluids. Certain specific chemicals show up in most patients with certain disease. Certain specific chemicals that is normally present in our body increases or decreases to certain levels in certain specific conditions in most of the patients. Please note that I am talking about "most patients" not "all patients". This point will be very important as we discuss more.

Medical knowledge about human diseases basically comes from observation or study of group of patients. All the data regarding the usefulness of these blood tests are also obtained from analysis of groups of patients- either passively observed or directly studied. If a certain chemical in the blood was found to be elevated in the majority of patients with certain diagnosis, then the blood test to determine the level of that chemical in the blood will be studied as a potentially useful blood test to make the diagnosis. Then that theory will be tested in other groups of patients and if the results are persistent, then that test will be used in clinical practice.

The interesting thing here is that even when a blood test is determined to be very useful, the results of the study will be surprising to you if you look at the details. There will always be some patients who had positive test but did not have the disease and there will always be patients who had negative tests and did have the disease. No matter how expensive or how technologically advanced equipment is used for the blood test, no single blood test or any other test in medicine is 100% accurate in predicting the presence or absence of a disease. Do not get me wrong here, the technology used in the lab is pure science, it is very accurate, and the lab has the capacity to very accurately measure the amount of that chemical in the blood. The inaccuracy lies in predicting the presence of the disease in an individual patient based on that test result.

If you are with me so far, I would like to explain to you a little bit further about the tests. Since all tests are imperfect, doctors usually like to know how imperfect the particular test is and they look at two different qualities of the test. The first thing they like to know is what percentage of the patients that have the disease will have positive test. This quality of the test is called the sensitivity of the test. If a test is 90% sensitive, it means that if 10 patients with that disease are tested, nine of them are likely to have a positive test. In other words, among the 10 patient, there will be one person who will be falsely labeled as negative and not having the disease who in fact does have it. In actual practice, if a test has a sensitivity of 90%, it is considered a very sensitive test. It means that based on these tests, one out of 10 diagnosis will be missed.

Scary, isn't it? Do not worry, please continue reading and you will be able to see the bigger picture.

Another quality of these imperfect tests that doctors like to know is called the specificity. It is the percentage of the patients correctly identified as not having the disease based on the test result. If the specificity of the test is 90% and there are 10 patients who do not have the disease, 9 of them will have a negative test result. Just like previously discussed, it also means that one patient who does not have the disease will be falsely identified as having the disease. And that means one out of ten patient will have a wrong diagnosis.

If you have been with me so far, you will find out that if the doctors made their decisions solely based on these so called highly accurate tests with a 90% sensitivity and 90% specificity, one out of ten patients will have a missed diagnosis and one out of ten patients will have a wrong diagnosis.

There are tests that are more sensitive but less specific and there are other tests which are less sensitive but very specific. Let me give you an interesting example from a real life scenario. You may have heard about the great fire that damaged the most of the city of Chicago years ago. If not, you may still have heard or seen a fire that has destroyed life and property. In general, there is a great fear of fire in our society. Billions of dollars are spent to prevent and fight fire in the United States every year. Fire fighters are considered American heroes as they are the protectors who save lives and properties from this most dreaded natural enemy. As a result, public policy makers do not want to miss any fire. They have therefore developed very sensitive smoke detectors to prevent fire. These are designed not to miss any fire at all.

If you happen to visit one specific high rise apartment building in Chicago, you will be surprised to see what happens there. If you are visiting a friend for dinner and are planning to spend your night there, chances are that you will hear the fire alarm go off at around dinner time. You will start panicking and will try to run to find the nearest fire escape and stairway. You will be very surprised to see that your friend is calm and seems unaffected as if she is deaf and has not heard the fire alarm at all. She continues to eat and does not even leave the dinner table. You find the fire exit, you find the stairway, you run down 30 flights of stairs and thank god you are out of the harms way. But, wait a minute, you do not see a big crowd coming out of the building. You wonder where the occupants of the building with more than 400 apartments went. You thought your friend was crazy for not leaving the dinner table after hearing the fire alarm. Could all these people have gone crazy too?

Well, here is what happened. There has not been an actual fire in that building. But people have been hearing fire alarms go off almost everyday. And now they stopped panicking about the fire alarm and even started to neglect it. How did this happen? Well, like I said fire alarm is designed to not miss any fire. In that sense they are designed to be very sensitive, almost 100% sensitive. It means that if there is a fire one hundred times, it will go off without defect in each case. The flip side is when you are making something that sensitive, it is very difficult to make it highly specific. It is designed to pickup even the tiniest bit of smoke. You can not design something that only detects real fire if you want it to be sensitive enough to pick up even the tiniest amount of smoke. What are the chances that one of 400 kitchens in the high rise has the cooking oil slightly overheated to produce a small amount of smoke? About 1 or 2 a day.

What would have happened if they had made that smoke detector 100% specific instead of 100% sensitive? Then the detector would not go off unless there was an actual fire. Let's say it was 100% specific and 99% sensitive. Sounds good enough? Well, let's see. A sensitivity of 99% means that it will pick up a real fire 99 times out of 100 fires. It also means that , it will miss one out of a hundred fires. With something as destructive as fire, is it good enough to detect it only 99% of the times? Most people would say no and I agree.

Well, why can't they make it 100% sensitive and 100% specific? Let's explore that. A smoke detector detects fire by analyzing the amount of smoke in the air. To be 100% sensitive, it has to detect even the slightest bit of smoke in the air so that it does not miss any fire. To be 100% specific, it has to go off only when there is enough smoke in the air that can be caused by an actual fire so that it does not "misdiagnose" normal cooking as fire. As you can see, the smoke detector can not have both. They have to choose one strength over the other and they rightly chose sensitivity over specificity. The disadvantage is that the firefighters have to make a trip to that building everyday and thousands of dollars are spent for the false alarm. As you will be reading in the next few chapters, this analogy goes very well in the way healthcare system functions in this county.

Most medical tests are in a way similar to the smoke detector. When our organs become damaged, they release certain chemicals in our blood in the same way smoke is released by a burning fire. But these chemicals may also be produced in small amounts in the body during normal metabolic activities in the same way small amount of smoke is produced during normal cooking. The exact amount of the chemical produced by the normal organ is slightly different in different individuals. If you put a low threshold for a positive test, there will be a few individuals with a normal organ producing just enough amount of chemical to labeled as abnormal. If you put the threshold too high, you will not mislabel any normal amount as abnormal but you may fail to detect some of the damaged ones.

You may be wondering how to trust this health care system where the tests are so imperfect: 1 in 10 disease is missed and 1 in 10 is misdiagnosed. That is where the art of medicine plays its parts. If all tests and treatments were perfect, doctors would be extinct and replaced by labs and computers. Unlike computers and labs, human brain has a higher but imperfect ability to look at the bigger picture and make intellectual and subjective analysis to try to recognize a pattern rather than make all decisions based on factual data and numbers. This unique human ability is an art and can not be replaced by machines. It is similar to the difference between a photograph and an artistic portrait. A portrait is made by an artist who does not draw her strokes by measuring the person with an inch tape, who does not use numbers and calculations to make an exact replica of the person. She lets her mind control her hand and draws as she sees. A portrait may not be an exact replica of a person but can do more than a picture can; it can capture and highlight emotions and

> It takes a doctor with an imperfect human brain to practice medicine in a world where the tests available to him are imperfect. A good doctor does not completely rely on these tests but uses the subjective information obtained from the patient to formulate his diagnosis. He tries to put everything together and attempts to know the patient as a person and only orders right tests in the right context so that the test results make more sense.

feelings.

It takes a doctor with an imperfect human brain to practice medicine in a world where the tools available to him are imperfect. This is the reason why a good doctor attempts to obtain as much subjective information from a patient as possible, not just the information related to the medical condition. He will attempt to explore your personal life, your family, your bad habits, your occupation and your educational level. He tries to know the patient as a person and explores and tries to put each symptom in the context of the patient's life and makes educated guess based on the available information. He does not completely rely upon the test results but use them as a guide to recognize the pattern and make the correct diagnosis. If, based on his subjective assessment and gut feeling, he thinks that a certain diagnosis is highly probable, he does not reject it just because the test came back negative.

Chapter 5: Why would anyone lie to the doctor?

How does the doctor find out what is wrong with you?

Well, basically — you tell him.

Yes, that is right. You just learned that in chapter 2. The most important source of information used in making the correct diagnosis is based on what the patient actually tells the doctor.

So what happens when you lie to the doctor?

> People do lie to their doctors and the doctors know that some of the patients lie to them but can not always tell when someone is lying. They always think about the possibility that the patient could be lying when presented with unusual symptoms. But they try to find some other possible explanations before entertaining that idea.

When people are frustrated, overwhelmed or under a lot of pressure, they sometimes do fake symptoms. Yes, some patients do fake symptoms and doctors know that some patients fake symptoms but are not always able to tell when someone is faking the symptoms the first time.

So, why do they fake symptoms? Sometimes the reason is obvious and easy to understand. You can think of a number of reasons someone you know might have faked symptoms — to avoid work, to avoid stressful situation, to get out of school, or sometimes even to try to get out of a traffic ticket. But there are times when the reason is much more complex and more difficult to understand.

Some of the patients are even themselves unaware that

they are faking the symptoms. Yes, that is true. Sometimes people are faking symptoms and are seeking medical attention, but they might themselves be unaware that their symptoms are not real. And then there are others who are in a different category. They do know that they are faking their symptoms and they keep doing it but do not know why they are doing it and also do not want to know why they are doing it.

So what happens when patients go to the doctors with fake symptoms? Shouldn't intelligent doctors with years of training and experience be able to detect these fake symptoms the moment they see them?

The reality is quite different. As explained in the earlier chapter, although the technology used in the medical treatment and diagnosis is very advanced, clinical medicine is still very subjective and primitive. More often than not, when such a patient is seen for the first time, the clinician is easily fooled and makes diagnosis based on the presenting symptoms.

When people are overwhelmed by life circumstances and are under a lot of stress, they might perceive their anxiety and depression as physical symptoms. When they are depressed and feeling low, they might believe they are having a "heart attack" when they are in fact having a panic attack. Of course ,in this society, it is easier to seek help for chest pain than it is for depression. It also gives the patient a false sense of security that the symptoms are from a physical illness and not a psychological one. They would feel much better if they believe that the problem is with their body and is not under with their mind. They start to believe that they do get chest pain and decide to go to seek help for the chest pain.

With a symptom like chest pain, the threshold to order more tests is very low. A heart attack can be fatal if not diagnosed early. Even when the presenting symptoms are not very convincing or typical for a heart attack, doctors always proceed with caution. There are always a fraction of patients whose description of chest pain is very atypical but end up having a real heart attack.

When that patient with the perceived chest pain is seen in the emergency room, she will most likely be admitted to the hospital, will be kept on a cardiac monitor. This will make the patient believe even more firmly that she is really sick. The fact that she was kept in the hospital and had close monitoring and given different medicines will leave a lasting and deep impression in that person's heart that something is definitely wrong with her. After the overnight observation, the patient will be discharged in the morning after all the tests are negative. At that time, she will be somewhat disappointed that all the tests are negative as this will be a challenge to her belief that she has a serious disease that is causing her to be distressed. It will be very difficult for her to even think that the distress is expressing itself as physical

> People who lie to the doctor basically fall into three categories. Some lie to the doctor for obvious secondary gain that is easy to understand. Others lie to the doctor but do not even know that they are lying. The other category of patients know that they are lying to the doctor but do not know why they have to lie but continue to do so.

symptoms. Her psychological defense mechanism will come up with a alternative explanation that will help her stay on her belief.

Instead of believing that her heart is normal, she will start to believe that she has something more serious that they were not able to find out in the hospital. In fact, our healthcare system's imperfections are perfect to lead her into such beliefs and re-confirm her convictions. As explained earlier, the diagnosis making process relies heavily on what the patient is actually telling you. And even the most sophisticated "stress test" used to diagnose heart disease is at most only 90% sensitive which means that 10% of the times it may miss a person with heart disease. There is a risk that 10% of patients who do happen to have heart disease will have a negative test result and will be discharged home. The doctor who is discharging this patient knows the limitations of test he just performed on the patient. In this situation when confronted by the patient with the question," Doctor, are you sure there is absolutely no problem with my heart?", the best reassuring answer he can give is: "With his negative stress test and the type of symptoms you have, the likelihood of any serious heart disease is very little." These words may be very reassuring to a hopeful regular patient who was hoping and praying for the test to be negative. But for the patient just described, it presents a hope, a hope that her symptoms could still be from her heart. She might want to reconfirm that suspicion by asking again: "Doctor, are you 100% sure that it is not my heart?" then the doctor has no option but to answer: "No I can not guarantee 100%, but…." She will stop hearing after that and block out the rest.

After this incident, the patient will start to have a fixed belief in her mind that something is wrong with her body and not with their mind. Some of them even take it to next level. They now start developing new symptoms every time they get depressed.

By this time she has been in and out of hospitals so many times that she has started to learn what symptoms will get the most attention and what symptoms trigger what tests. She has now learned to express her symptoms in a way that draws the most attention of the doctors and nurses. As time goes by, she becomes so perfect that a doctor who sees for the first time might be convinced that she does have a real heart disease. As the most important information required to make a diagnosis is what she tells the doctor, the doctor might diagnose her with heart disease despite the negative test result. This can happen because the doctor can not always rely on the test when the story the patient gives is very convincing. He knows that the test does not always come back positive in all patients with heart disease.

Finally, her prayers are answered. She somehow found the doctor that is also convinced that she has a heart disease. Finally, she feels as if someone has found the root cause of all her misery.

Now she will be having an invasive procedure for the first time. She will be taken to an operating room. What she does not understand is that what she is about to have is a real medical procedure that was not necessary. She will be signing papers where she understands that there can be life threatening complications from the procedure itself.

There is a reason why this procedure is only performed in patients who have a very high chance of actually having a heart disease capable of possibly killing them. The suspicion of life threatening heart disease should be so high that the risk of dying from the procedure is actually considered an acceptable risk. But for our patient, none of those matters. She is so excited to be under the doctor's knife that she signs all the warning and consent papers happily with a hope that all her misery will be gone.

If she gets lucky, she will go through the procedure without any complications. She will be somewhat disappointed that her heart is normal but she will still be satisfied by the fact that she has achieved a significant milestone. She had the right symptoms that triggered a trip to the operating room. The important thing here to remember is that she is doing all of this subconsciously. She believes that the physical symptoms that she is producing in herself is real. She believes she is miserable because of these medical problems. To think that she is miserable because of her depression or because of other life circumstances is exactly what her mental defense mechanism is trying to avoid.

After the procedure is done and she comes back again with the same symptom, the doctor starts to get a little skeptical. With all the typical symptoms, negative stress test and even a normal invasive test, now the doctor begins to think. Could this be somehow related to her depression? But that is a big step to consider. Once you begin to think in that way about your patient, you begin to question the authenticity of your patient's symptom. This can be very challenging. When he tries to ask the patient about depression and any life stresses, she becomes disappointed. Suddenly the great doctor is not great anymore. She gets upset, goes home, pulls herself together and next week when she has the symptoms again, she decides to go to a new doctor.

If the new doctor is able to obtain medical records from the previous doctor, he will send her home if she comes back with a chest pain. She goes home disappointed but still has a hope that they could find something wrong with her body. After the first few visits, she is disappointed that the new doctor seems to be ignoring her chest pain. At that time, she suddenly "finds out" that her abdomen also hurts. With the new symptom of abdominal pain, she is once again able to get adequate attention from the doctors and the nurses. After she is sent home for her abdominal pain a few times, she will start to learn what type of abdominal pain gets the most attention. If she learns it right, she will have the type of abdominal pain that is bad enough to convince the doctor that she needs a surgery. In this way, she may actually have a few abdominal surgeries during the next few years.

After a few abdominal surgeries that did not reveal any pathology, she might develop a headache. Now she will learn to "have" headaches associated with blurry vision which buys her an overnight hospital stay with close monitoring.

After seven or eight years of numerous doctor visits, two cardiac catheterizations, one gall bladder surgery, two additional abdominal surgeries, multiple hospitalizations and a medical record as thick as an encyclopedia, she is still convinced that she has multiple medical problems that are causing all her life distress. At this time, she visits a new doctor for a new problem. When he reviews all her medical problems, one thing will strike him as quite unusual. All the procedures, all the tests have been normal despite these years of complicated and complex symptoms. Even the gall bladder that was removed did not have any signs of inflammation. This time, for the first time, the doctor will start to suspect the real diagnosis " Munchhausen syndrome". Yes, this is a real disease and real diagnosis and a one that is very difficult and daring to make. This is how a patient with this syndrome presents in reality in our health care system. Most of the practicing physicians would have taken care of patients with this syndrome at some point in their practice. Some would have never even realized that they had taken care of one. This is a psychological disorder which causes the patients to fake, develop and exaggerate symptoms without any conscious secondary gain from it. At an unconscious level, the patient is trying to blame her body for the trouble her mind is having. As the disease progresses, she starts to enjoy the medical procedures and the attention she gets in the hospital. The uncertainties and imperfections of the modern medicine and the medical tests play a big role in how these patients go undetected for many years. During this time, most of them get actual medical problems as a result of complication from one of the procedures that they have received over the years.

Yes, sad but true.

Chapter 6: My niece is a nurse.

I do not go to my doctor without her. She can really explain things to my doctor. She is my greatest asset.

Congratulations for having a nurse in your family. Yes, she is your big asset. You must be very proud of her. It is normal to feel somewhat anxious during a doctor's visit. After all, you are getting information about the most important thing in your life — you health. You are also anxious that you might forget to ask the right question and also that you might miss any pertinent information that you need to tell your doctor. In these moments, you feel that you would wish there was someone with you who could speak for you. You wish there was someone asking questions to the doctor for you. You wish you had someone that can understand the medical terms for you. In other words, you wish there was someone to advocate for you with your doctor in the same way your lawyer advocates for you when you are dealing with a legal matter. You find that your niece fits the bill perfectly. You saw her grow up. You love her. She loves you. She cares for you. She is your perfect girl. You are her favorite aunt. You were very proud when she went to the nursing school. Now she is a practicing nurse. She has been working alongside doctors. She shares her interesting stories with you. She knows the medical field. Now you have a real medical advocate for you.

Well, most of the times, it is very good to have such a personal medical advocate in your family. It helps you to remain motivated to get all the tests done, have regular doctor visits, take your medications and be more proactive in maintaining your health.

Now, lets discuss what could happen when you are not feeling well. Naturally, you would call your niece before calling the doctor. Your niece will visit with you. She will try to find out if you really need to go to the hospital or not. She might check your blood pressure if she has a machine at home. If she finds out that your blood pressure is high, she will take you to the hospital. By the time she has reached the hospital with you, she will have discussed your symptoms in detail and she has some ideas about what could be wrong and what tests need to be done. At the same time, you are very reassured that your niece is with you and that she understands your symptoms and she knows what needs to be done. Up to this point, everything is reasonable and she has really been very helpful.

When the doctor finally sees you, your niece is with you. Whenever he asks you questions, you naturally turn towards your niece and expect her to answer the questions for you. By now, you feel like she knows more about what is happening with you than you do. But the doctor is interested in hearing what you have to say — not how your niece interprets your symptoms. The scenario can get very frustrating for the doctor who does not really want to offend your niece but is trying his best to get a good description of events from you. But, you feel that how you felt is less important and the most important thing is to get the things that your niece wants done for you.

Doctor: "What is the reason you are here today"

You: "My niece here is a nurse and she checked me out and knew right away that I needed to come to the hospital."

Doctor: "And why is that?"

You: "You ask her. She is the nurse. She knows the medical stuff."

Doctor: "But what was the reason you had to call her?"

You: "Why? I always call her when I need help. She takes good care of me. I am proud of her."

Doctor: "I am interested in knowing how you felt or what happened to you that you had to call your niece."

My niece is a nurse.

You: "Oh, my blood pressure was high. That's what she told me. That's why I am here. Now she wants to make sure I did not have a heart attack"

Doctor: "But what did you feel that made you think you might have a heart attack?"

You: "How do I know? I am not a nurse, she is."

If you read chapter 2, you can probably understand the frustration the doctor can have by the conversation so far. He has not been able to get any important information about the patient's symptoms that would help him make the diagnosis. The doctor is interested in what actually happened to you and how you felt when your symptoms started.

At this point the doctor has no choice but to turn to your niece for more questions. There is no harm in asking your niece about what happened to you but it is not as helpful as the first hand subjective information that you could have given the doctor yourself. Another problem in this approach is that because she is a nurse, she has already processed the information with her medical knowledge and already has a theory about what could have happened. In that case, her memory will be somewhat biased by what she thinks is going on with her Aunt. If she thought that her aunt was having a heart attack, she will selectively remember the things that would go along with the diagnosis of a heart attack. But the doctor wants to evaluate the chest pain with an open mind. He wanted to know how exactly it started, where it went from there , how exactly the patient felt when she had the pain. He wanted to first evaluate which organ the pain might be coming from before jumping to the diagnosis. He wanted to see if it could

> It is good to have your own healthcare advocate in your family. But unlike your legal advocate, there are situations where you should speak for yourself in regards to your symptoms to help the doctor find the right diagnosis.

be from her lungs instead of her heart. He wanted to know if there were certain qualities of the pain that would make him suspect that it could be actually from one of the big blood vessels in the neck instead of the heart itself.

By pointing to your niece as a proxy for your healthcare, you are missing this great opportunity to help your doctor find the right diagnosis for you. The result would be that because of the pre-processed information, your doctor will be forced to think in the same direction that your nurse was thinking and that can sometimes lead to an important diagnosis being missed.

You knew that having a healthcare advocate for you in your family is very good for you but now you probably understand that there are some situations when it is best that you speak for yourself. That may not be true in regards to your legal advocate but it is true regarding your healthcare advocate.

Chapter 7: What can the doctor find out just by listening with the stethoscope?

This piece of equipment has been associated with medical practice for so long that any mental picture of a doctor is incomplete without a stethoscope hanging down his shoulder. To a patient, nothing gives more reassurance than knowing that the doctor just listened to their chest with the stethoscope and everything sounded OK. In this chapter, we will explore what information can be obtained by listening to your chest with the stethoscope and how much and in what situation that information helps the doctor to make the correct diagnosis. We will also be exploring what other methods of this process called physical exam are employed by the doctor to help make your diagnosis.

You probably know that the stethoscope is a listening equipment. You probably guessed it as it goes into the doctor's ears. So, what exactly is the doctor listening for? Before we go into this, let's explore what is the main goal of a complete physical exam and how it is done.

In fact, the physical exam actually starts at the time when the doctor is talking to you. When you are talking to the doctor, he is not only listening to what you are saying but he is also listening to the quality of your voice and looking for any abnormality in the sound of your voice. He is also evaluating the content of your speech to make sure that what you are saying is actually in agreement with what is going on at that movement. When talking to the patient, the doctor is not only conducting the medical history but is also starting his physical exam. The doctor tries to use all five senses while conducting a physical exam to try to collect clues about the state of your internal organs.

The first part of the physical exam is called inspection and observation. This seems to be an obvious and easy step but it can easily give your doctor a very important information that will help nail the correct diagnosis. It can be as important as listening to your chest in obtaining the correct diagnosis. General inspection includes an overall assessment to see how “sick” the patient looks. The doctor will be looking for signs of distress when evaluating the degree of sickness. If the patient appears lethargic, sweaty or has trouble speaking because of sickness, that patient needs prompt attention as these are signs that the patient's body is in imminent danger and has been overwhelmed. On the other hand, if someone is shouting and screaming and demanding to be seen right away, that person may appear to be more distressed to the common eyes but not necessarily to the doctor's eyes. Of the two patients just described, the doctor will always focus his attention to the first one. The second patient is agitated but not necessarily distressed. Most of the times, patients who are really distressed are too tired to be shouting and screaming.

After general inspection, the next step is to note the vital signs. These are some numbers and measurements that represent the basic state of your body at that particular time. There are four basic measurements that are considered to be the most basic indicators of bodily function. The first one is the body temperate which is measured with a thermometer and is recorded in degrees Fahrenheit in US and degrees Centigrade in some other countries. This tells the doctor if you are having a fever. We all know high temperature is abnormal and indicates fever. Low temperature is also abnormal and is called hypothermia.

The next vital sign is the pulse or the heart rate. It is measured either by counting your pulsation in your wrist or by actually listening to your heart-beat. This number not only gives the state of your heart-beat but also gives an overall assessment of the stress your body is under. Very high or very low pulse represents severe distress and imminent danger.

After the pulse, the next vital sign is the respiratory rate. It is obtained by simply counting how many times you are breathing in one minute. The respiratory rate can change just based on your anxiety level as you tend to breathe fast when you are anxious. At the same time, high respiratory rate can also be a signal that your breathing is highly stressed. The doctor will look for other signs of distress when evaluating a high respiratory rate to determine it's significance.

The other vital sign is the blood pressure. There are several different ways of measuring blood pressure and one of the methods needs the use of a stethoscope. But, most of the times it is measured with an automated machine in most US hospitals. It gives an estimate of the pressure created by the flow of your blood inside your blood vessels. Blood pressure is not a constant number but fluctuates significantly according to the time of the day, state of your mind, your bodily stress and other factors. Too high or too low blood pressure needs prompt management in the right context.

> The stethoscope is a listening device that transmits sounds from the surface of the body to the doctor's ears. The only organs that produce audible sound are the ones with the moving parts.

After the general inspection and vital signs, the doctor moves on to the specific organ system examination. In this process, he will examine each organ using the same principal that he used for the general exam. He will attempt to use all his senses to try to detect any abnormalities. He will look, feel, press, listen and percuss as necessary to detect any variations from normal. This organ system exam can be very brief if the doctor is just looking for a particular organ system disease or can be a detailed one if he is considering a number of different possibilities.

The stethoscope is used for the listening part of the body organ system exam. It is therefore only a small part of the complete physical exam. It is simply an instrument that transmits sound from your body surface to the doctor's ears. Not all body organs make sound. The only organs that produce audible sounds are the ones that have moving parts. The most important of these is your heart. The other organs that have significant movement are the lungs, the stomach and the intestines. Sometimes, large blood vessels can also make enough sound from the movement of the blood that can be heard with the stethoscope.

When the doctor puts the stethoscope on the front mid section of your chest, he is listening to your heart-beat. At this point, it is not necessary to take deep breaths. Heart is a pump that pumps your blood to the whole body. Just like any other pump, it needs valve mechanisms to function if you want the blood to flow in a certain direction. Just like the heat pump in your furnace or the water pump in your pool, the heart also makes some sound when it is operating. If you hear an abnormally loud sound from your furnace pump, you worry that the pump might be failing or malfunctioning. In a similar way, the doctor worries about a failing heart pump if he hears abnormal sounds in your heart. But a malfunctioning pump does not always make abnormal sound and not all abnormal sounds indicate pump malfunction. This is equally true with your heart. There are normal variability in heart sounds in different individual depending on the age, sex, chest muscle and other factors.

The most common abnormal sound detected with the stethoscope is called a heart murmur. It is the sound transmitted by the heart valves. They are produced by leaky valves or valves that are too tight. But not all heart murmurs are abnormal. Sometimes, a little bit of leaking and a little bit of tightness may be within normal limits.

The more important fact about the heart sounds is that you can have a very serious heart disease and you may not have any abnormal sound with it. Only a small fraction of patients with a heart attack have an abnormal heart sound. When your doctor is evaluating your chest pain, an abnormal heart sound will give the doctor very important piece of information but a normal heart sound does not provide any reassurance at all.

When the doctor puts the stethoscope on the back and the sides of your chest, he is listening to your lung sounds. It is this part of the exam that the doctor asks you to take deep breaths. Your heart beats automatically and is not under your control. But the movement of your lungs can be under your control. You can voluntarily control how deep or how fast you want to take your breaths. Unlike the heart, the lungs only make sounds when the air is going in and out of your lungs. If you hold your breath for a while, the doctor will not be hearing any sound from your lungs.

The two most common types of abnormal lung sounds are called crackles and wheezing. Crackles are produced when there is fluid present in the air tubes of your lungs. When air travels through these fluids, it makes a crackly sound. When the air pipes are too narrow, the air traveling through these pipes make a whistle like sound called wheezing. This is very common in patients with asthma. Again, abnormal sounds are not always heard with all lung diseases and not all abnormal lung sounds are associated with lung disease.

> Listening with a stethoscope is only a small part of this process called physical exam. The doctor tries to examine the signals transmitted by your internal organs using all his senses during the physical exam. Abnormal findings in the physical exam help the doctor in making diagnosis but normal findings may not provide any reassurance.

Besides the heart and the lungs, the other places the doctor normally listens to is the abdomen. Here, he listens to the sounds produced by the moving intestines and stomach. The stomach and intestines are always in motion but the amount of motion depends on different factors. Absent or very sluggish sound is abnormal and warrants further investigation. Very high pitched and overactive sounds can also be abnormal.

The other use of the stethoscope is to listen for the fetal heart-beat in a pregnant patient but this use has mostly been replaced by the ultrasound machines these days.

Chapter 8: My friend just died from ovarian cancer.

Why do they not test every woman for ovarian cancer just like they do for breast cancer?

Prevention is better than cure, right? The earlier you can detect the risk factors for a disease, the better you can prevent that disease by controlling the risk before it becomes a problem. With today's technology, many diseases can be detected early before they cause any symptom. But we still hear about cases of lung cancers diagnosed "too late" to be cured. Thousands of women

> We hear about the sad stories of many women who eventually die from ovarian cancer every year. Most of them had been told that it was too late at the time of the diagnosis. After hearing these stories, it is only natural to think that we should be testing every healthy women for ovarian cancer just like we do for breast cancer.

still die from ovarian cancer every year. If you search the internet for ovarian cancer, you will find numerous heart breaking stories written by women diagnosed with ovarian cancer. Most of them are told,"It was too late." They were left with great resentment that nothing was done to detect it early. They have been urging the women and the society to take action. This topic has widespread discussion in the media and some have even advocated public policy change encouraging screening for ovarian cancer.

Then, why are they not doing it? When a woman reads that story and goes to her doctor and asks why is her doctor not screening her for ovarian cancer, how can that doctor defend himself? Is it a failure of our health care system? Is it a really bad practice? Should we demand congress to take action and should all women go to Capitol Hill to demonstrate and demand action? After all, it is about women's health and it is about saving life.

Let's explore how screening works. When you screen for a disease, you are looking to identify some indicator that will tell you that certain disease process has actually started in your body but it is too early for any symptoms to appear. There are thousands of human diseases and millions of medical tests designed to detect or diagnose these diseases. With this in mind, if the goal is to detect any disease before it starts expressing its symptoms, it seems like a very good idea to run these tests on everyone so that we can detect every disease very early and start treating before it gets out of hand. At this point, it seems logical to run a series of blood tests, CT scans, PET scans and MRI scans on everyone at least once a year if that will help detect diseases early and save lives.

Now let's look at it from a different point of view. Lets say, you are a professional woman in your thirties. You are very successful in your career. You have a great loving family. You go for a regular health screening as a benefit of your new exciting career. Let's say, ovarian cancer screening has been advocated by the media based on the heart-breaking stories from women who have died from it. You doctor offers you a blood test and a ultrasound to screen for ovarian cancer.

If you read my previous chapters, you probably know that medical tests are not perfect. There will always be times when the test results are abnormal in patients without actual disease. It means than there will be patients that will be labeled as having a positive test, even though they do not have the disease. Unfortunately, you happen to fall in that category. You have a falsely elevated blood test or some artifact seen in your ovaries. Now suddenly, your life has been changed. Instead of focusing on your new exciting job, now you have a huge burden to fight. You are scared for your life, you have been told that you have a test that indicates you might have an ovarian cancer.

Now you will go back and read the same stories that

prompted the media to advocate screening for ovarian cancer in the first place. You will be so worried by the stories about how their lives were changed by the diagnosis and what these women had to go through in their life. You will be seeing all these things happening in your life. This will be so devastating for you that you will have a very hard time focusing on your job. At the same time, you now have a higher pressure to keep your job as you now have a "pre-condition" which makes it very difficult for you to be able to get any private health insurance coverage if you loose your job.

You will eventually be cleared off the suspicion but that will not come easy. When someone is screened positive for possible ovarian cancer, it is taken very seriously.

It takes a lot of work and confidence to tell someone:"No, you do not have ovarian cancer, that test was likely false."

"And how did you come to that conclusion?"

" By doing another test."

"And how accurate is this another test?"

"More accurate than the first one."

Just like every test can have false positive result, it also can have false negative result.

"If you are saying that the first test was false positive, how do you know that the second test was not a false negative?"

The only way to do that is to make sure the second test is much more specific than the first test. And usually, it means that the test will be more expensive and often more invasive.

For example, the first test was an ultrasound which showed something in the ovaries that looked a little bit suspicious for an ovarian cancer. The only way to find out if that "shadow" on the ultrasound is cancer is to actually get a needle into that ovary, get a piece of it and send it for testing under the microscope to see if it actually contains cancer cells. In some specific cases, even that might not be enough. The result of the needle guided surgery may be equivocal and they may have to surgically remove that ovary to make the final diagnosis.

At other times, the second test will show that it is most likely not ovarian cancer but they can not be 100% sure.

"What do I do then?"

"Come back in 6 weeks to get another ultrasound."

Now, you will be anxious and fearful for weeks. You are not able to devote your mind to your family or your job. You will be anxiously waiting, having nightmares, reading about ovarian cancer and getting more and more withdrawn from your work and family in the coming weeks. During this time, you could actually develop anxiety and depression severe enough to require medication.

You could even lose your job because of the stress and inability to focus on your work. With a job loss, you could even lose your health insurance coverage. Finally after months of testing and even possible surgical biopsy, you will be told that you did not actually have cancer. It was just a "cyst" or some other harmless condition that looked like a cancer on the first test.

This side of the screening for a disease does not get discussed anywhere outside the doctor's conference room or the board of public health policy makers.

You may now be wondering: "Why do they still do regular screening for so many diseases if screening itself can cause so much harm?" There are a lot of different factors that need to be considered to decide which disease is suitable for screening.

The first criteria the disease has to meet is that it must be a relatively common disease. When we say relatively common, a number like one in one hundred to one in one thousand or sometimes even up to one in ten thousand is considered relatively common from a public health point of view. If a disease occurs only about one in a million or one in one hundred thousand, it may not be suitable for screening. This is relatively easy to understand. If a disease only happens to one person in a population of one million, then if you screen for the disease, you will be testing about one million people before you actually find one person that actually has the disease.

This is not to say that one life in a crowd of one million is not significant. Let us explore what could happen if we actually decide to screen one million people. Let us assume, we have a very accurate test that we can use to do the screening. Let's say this test is 99% sensitive and 99% specific.

Let's try this in a population of one million. If the test is 99% specific, we will have one false positive in one hundred tests. In a population of one million, we will have ten thousand false positive results. But we know that the disease is so rare that

> The testing for a disease in all members of a population is called disease screening. There are certain characteristics of a disease that determine if that particular disease is suitable for screening. Sometimes, disease screening can have unintended bad consequences.

only one in one million will actually have it. But, all ten thousand people are under severe stress to know that they might have this very rare disease. The only way to move ahead would be to do more tests on all these people to be able to find out which one of them actually has the disease. Until then, all ten thousands of them will be assumed to have it and are treated the same. After a series of more invasive, more complicated and more expensive tests, you will finally find the one person that you intended to help with all the tests that you did so far. Now, that would have been worth it if you had been able to do all the tests without causing any harm to other people. But when ten thousand people undergo invasive testing, the chances are that some of them may have bad complications from the tests.

Having said that, there are actually a very few diseases

where you can test a large number of people to identify one patient without doing much harm to the rest of them. One such disease is called Phenylketonuria and happens in about one in fifteen thousand to one in one hundred thousand depending on the race and geographical location. The screening test for this disease is done in everyone born across the United States. It is done right after birth by a simple blood test. The diagnosis is quick and does not cause any harm. If diagnosed at birth, treatment can be started right away and it saves a lot of trouble in the future.

The next important thing to consider in making decision about screening for a particular disease is the availability of suitable tests for that particular disease. Without a reliable and accurate test, it will be very difficult to perform any screening. For the test to be useful, it must be very sensitive, which means that it should be able to detect maximum number of people that have the disease. If it only picks up a fraction of people, then it will not be a useful screening test. But we know that if you design the test to be able to pick up most of the diseased patient, it will also pick up a few normal people by mistake. Now for a effective screening strategy, you need a set of tests. Like I explained earlier, the first test needs to be very sensitive. After you have selected the group of people with positive test results from the screening test, you will need a second test called the confirmatory test. Like the name implies, the confirmatory test must be a highly specific test. With the confirmatory test, you should be able to exclude all the normal people that have been wrongly labeled positive by the screening test.

The other requirement is that there has to be a very effective treatment for the disease if detected early. If we do not have a effective treatment, then there is no point in spending time and effort to detect the disease in its early stage. A very good example of this category of disease is breast cancer. Most breast cancer can be easily cured if it is diagnosed early. If discovered only in the late stage, breast cancer can be deadly. Breast cancer is also an example of a disease that has been extensively studied in regards to potential benefit from screening and is one of the few diseases that have proven screening benefits. They have clearly shown that breast cancer screening has saved lives.

The next thing to consider is called "the latent stage" of the disease. When people get a disease that has a latent stage, the disease will progress in several stages. In the first stage, people already have the disease but do not have any symptoms from it. This stage is called the latent stage of the disease. If a disease does not have a latent stage and starts to produce symptoms right away, then there is no need for the screening. The patient will present to the doctor with symptoms from the disease and will have medical evaluation done for diagnosis and treatment. Screening is only done in people that do not have any symptom of the disease yet.

By the time this book is written, I do not know of any highly sensitive screening test that has been shown to be beneficial in screening for ovarian cancer. There is also no effective confirmatory test that is specific enough to exclude the diagnosis in patients that are screened positive by the screening test. It does not mean that there will not be some tests in the future that could effectively be used for a good screening strategy in preventing deaths from ovarian cancer. But until then, you should know that you may get into a lot of unexpected problems if you decide to get tested for ovarian cancer when you do not have any symptoms from it.

But if you have a very high risk of ovarian cancer because of family history or because of some other factors, then the potential benefits of having the screening may outweigh the potential risks in your particular case. But that process is called selective screening of high risk patients. The scenario I described earlier applies to universal screening or screening of all women.

The purpose of this chapter is to give you an introduction about the potential harmful effects of screening. The decision to have screening test for any particular disease is your personal decision and only you and your doctor can decide if your circumstances warrant any screening test.

Chapter 9: You must be a genius to survive medical school, right?

That seems to be the perception of the public. Physicians are regarded as highly intellectual members of the society and parents assume that their children must be very intelligent to be able to survive medical school. Finishing medical school is considered by most to be an achievement of students with higher than average IQ. And most people think that higher the intelligence level of a doctor, the more successful he will be.

But the reality is that hard work and attention to details are the most important predictors of success in the medical career — far more important that high intelligence. Meticulous attention to details and working step by step with great patience is the best way to deliver good patient care and avoid mistakes. It is also very important to keep an open mind and not jump to conclusions too early. All of these tasks do not require higher than average intelligence. Medicine is definitely not one of those careers where higher intelligence gives you an edge to success. Higher intelligence is certainly rewarding in a profession that requires creativity, innovation and invention such as developers of new computer language or scientists in advanced physics working for NASA. Medicine is definitely not one of those subjects. Perseverance, compassion and meticulousness are more important than creativity, innovation and invention in the clinical medical career. Those who are more innovative than meticulous tend to go into medical research rather than clinical medicine.

The early years of medical school involves learning all about how human body functions. I am in no way implying that it is an easy task. I am only stating that you do not need to be a rocket scientist to learn these. What you need is deep and true interest in the human body and lots of hard work and persistence.

You have to learn how two hundred and eight pieces of bones are structured together to form the framework for the human body. You have to learn how each of these bones have different necks and curves to attach different muscles. You have to learn how contraction of which muscle turns which part of the body in which direction. You will have to learn what part of your brain has to send what specific signal to contract that particular muscle. You will have to learn what happens to the food you eat. You have to track every single inch in the path of the food which travels about thirteen meters inside your body before being excreted in your stool. You will have to understand how that food is broken down and what chemical reactions occur each step of the way. You will have to learn what happens to the air that you breathe inside your lungs. You will have to learn how your kidneys filter your blood and make urine. These tasks can be very overwhelming but anyone with a willingness to work hard can learn them. Anyone who can learn to be a car repair mechanic can learn to understand how a human body works. It is all about structure and function. There is a no abstract concept involved. There is no advanced calculus involved. There is no Einstein's theory of relativity involved.

The next important skill to survive medical school is to learn to avoid fear and aversion of things related to human body. Some students who went into medical school thinking about social prestige and glory of being a physician get very frustrated when they can not learn how to control their fear and aversion to certain things. Things that you should learn to avoid fear and aversion in medical school include dead body, rotten corpse, human feces, human urine, human blood or any other type of human secretion. When your job is to learn and master every nook and corner of the human body, you can not do that if you are averted by these things. There is no evidence that you need higher than average intelligence to be able to avoid the aversion to urine, feces and corpse.

The first few years of medical school can also be a time of great impatience. Everyday you keep thinking about when you will be able to see and examine actual patient instead of a corpse or a mannikin. This impatience can be quite frustrating and can derail you from your most important task on hand: learning to understand how human body works. At this point, there are always a few students who drop out and take a short route to actually start helping patients. They will find that becoming a paramedic or EMT better suits their personality. EMT and paramedics are very important part of the medical team and probably save more lives everyday than doctors do. But they do not need the depth of knowledge that medical students are required to acquire.

Finally when it is time for the most awaited clinical rotations during the latter years of medical school, they get a glimpse of the real world. By this time, they have mastered the knowledge of how human body works and how different disease

> Patience, perseverance, compassion,meticulousness and hard work are more important than intelligence, innovation and invention to succeed in medical school

process affect different organs and how different drugs work to treat different diseases. At this time, they are so confident that they believe they can diagnose and treat every patient they encounter.

But that confidence is usually very short lived. As soon as they start seeing real patients, they will start to know the difference between the human body they studied and the real human patient in front of them. So far they have mastered the "human body" not the "human patient". They will soon realize that real human patients are far more complex than the human body they have studied. They will start to notice that only using the textbook knowledge of medical facts do not solve the problems of the real human patient. Now they will finally begin to understand why medicine is a combination of art and science and not just a pure science. They will slowly learn that interpersonal skills, compassion, politeness and ability to remain calm under pressure are as important as medical knowledge in helping the real patient. It is normally during this phase of the medical training that most medical students decide what kind of doctor they want to be. At this stage, they will be working alongside actual doctors and real patients. They will also notice that not all doctors follow the textbook completely. They also notice how different doctors treat the same disease differently. They will slowly start to understand that there are different ways of doing things and there are more than one correct answers in the real world unlike the only one correct answer they have been sticking with so far for their medical school exams. They will also start to understand how patient's belief's, culture and life experience has to considered in making the right decision for the patient. At this point, they will also start to learn that what you believe is the best treatment for the patient may not always the best option for the patient.

How well a medical student learned the basic medical science of the human body in the first half of the medical school will determine how well that student may do on the standardized tests and board exams. But how well the future doctor does in his medical career and how happy and satisfied he will be as a doctor depends on how he learned the art of medicine during the latter half of his medical education.

Chapter 10: Half of what they teach in medical school is wrong. Can you believe it?

Believe it or not, half of what they teach in medical school is wrong. Does that disturb you? Well, here is a more disturbing fact — the medical school graduates do not know which half is wrong until about ten years after graduation.

If you do not believe me, you can go to any public library and find a standard medical textbook. First, find the current edition and just read one chapter. Now, ask the librarian to find the same textbook but an edition that was written ten years ago and read it. You will be surprised to find the difference. What was taught to be a factual treatment option ten years ago in a medical school is totally unaccepted today and is replaced by a different treatment modality. If you read all the chapters, you will find that only half of the knowledge in the textbook has remained the same after ten years. The medical student who graduated ten years ago could not have predicted which half would still be true ten years later.

> Because of the rapidly evolving nature of diagnostic methods, new treatment drugs and constantly changing nature of human diseases, what is taught in medical school now as undeniable factual knowledge will become only half true in just a few years from now. There is no way of predicting which half will still be true.

You can argue that things are different now, medical science is much more advanced and what we know now are all facts. But the student who graduated ten years ago would have thought the same if he had looked up an earlier edition, one ten years before him. If you practice medicine today based on what you learned ten years ago in medical school, that would be considered malpractice and yes you can loose your license. On the other hand, it is more interesting to note that if you were a real genius and able to see future and practiced medicine ten years ago based on what is acceptable now, you would still be convicted with malpractice.

But why is this happening? Shouldn't they be doing a better job at the medical school and teaching the right things?

Well, they are doing a good job. The problem is that the field of medical knowledge is constantly evolving. There is new information coming out from medical research everyday. What is considered a standard and acceptable practice today may no longer be acceptable one year from now.

The interesting point here is that the change in practice pattern is not always because of a better alternative that is now available. Sometimes, it is the opposite. Medical research not only finds out what new treatment options are better but it also finds out what we have been doing wrong. For example, they might discover a new miraculous drug that does wonders and cures previously incurable disease. Subsequently, that drug is used widely for many years. It is only after all these years that they seem to notice that people who were on these new drugs were actually having many serious problems that had not been noticed before these drugs became widely circulated. In certain circumstances, they might find out that the new medicine was causing more harm than help. In that case, we may need to go back to the previous drug that we had been using before the discovery of the so called miraculous new drug.

If you consider the rapidly growing number of drugs and diagnostic techniques that become available each year, it is not very difficult to believe that half of what is considered a fact now will no longer be true ten years later. We can again argue that we know more and more every year, a time will eventually come when we know everything and we will not be teaching anything wrong in the medical school anymore. Because of the methods of modern medicine and the nature of human diseases, that is not very likely to happen in at least the next two hundred years. That statement may seem like a very grave assessment of the progress that we have made in the medical field in the 21st century but you may understand the logic behind it after reading the whole chapter.

One factor interesting to note about medicine and diseases is that as we make progress in treating diseases, diseases themselves are evolving in a way that eventually requires new treatment. As we conquer one old disease another new disease appears and challenges us. This is especially true with regards to infectious diseases.

Diseases that are caused by bugs that infect different organ systems of the human body are classified as infectious disease. In the history of medicine, there have been many diseases that were at different times considered untreatable. We simply did not have any drug strong enough to kill that particular bug at that particular time. Patients who were infected with those bugs had no cure. With advancement in medical science, eventually drugs were discovered that were capable of killing those bugs and curing the disease. That was a great victory of mankind over that particular disease. Many lives were saved and many deaths prevented, many sufferings relieved. But while we were celebrating our victory over bugs, some of the bugs were not quite ready to accept the defeat. With multiple and widespread use of the same drugs, the few surviving bugs were working hard to develop a strategy to fight us back. How do they do that?

That is an interesting question. Well, they can take their chance. At least initially, "chance" plays a big part. Of the millions of bugs treated with the medicine, one of them somehow survives the attack. How does that happen? Well, mainly by chance. That is the lucky bug. Maybe he was made slightly differently than the rest of them. Maybe he had one of his organs missing. Maybe he was a handicapped bug and lacked the ability to perform certain bug functions. But this could be his lucky day. It could be that the exact organ or the exact function that bug was missing was the actual target of the drug. That drug would use that function or that organ to get inside the body of the bug to kill him. Now his disability is his blessing.

This lucky bug eventually starts to produce more bugs like himself. If you remember high school biology, you can probably recall that these bugs do not need a partner and do not need to have sex to reproduce. They can simply cut themselves into two halves and each half can grow up to become two young bugs. And when they mature, they too cut themselves into halves and become more young bugs. In this way, one bug becomes two, two become four and four become eight. In this way, after a few generations, one single bug can create a colony of bugs. In this case, one handicapped bug resistant to the drug can create an army of bugs that all have the power to fight back against that drug. And as time goes by, they are able to produce sufficient resistant bug. These bugs can thrive again and start causing disease again. They will not be touched by the drug that used to kill them. If doctors do not spot this phenomenon early and send the bugs to be tested for any resistance that is being developed, we will soon lose the battle against disease causing bugs. In fact, scientists and doctors around the world are constantly working to develop new drugs and modify old drugs to keep up with the resistance development process that the bugs are using constantly to fight back against our drugs. This is a battle between the mankind and the disease causing bugs that we can not afford to loose.

Now, let's go back to the medical school. Ten years ago the original drug was killing all of one particular type of bugs. For the disease caused by that bug, the drug was the considered the life saving miraculous drug. Ten years later, if the doctor who went to that medical school uses the same drug to treat the same disease, that drug would not touch these bugs and the patient may die from overwhelming infection.

So, how do doctors practice good medicine when they are taught so badly in the medical school?

You may think that medical education is complete when you graduate from a medical school. In fact, medical school is only the beginning of your medical education. It is not the end. Every single day after graduation from the medical school is a whole new chapter in your medical education. Medical education only ends when you retire from your medical career. Graduating from medical school is only like mastering the alphabets of medicine. Without mastering the alphabets, you can not learn the language. But at the same time, you can not master a language by just knowing the alphabets. You have to go out and start reading. Similarly, in medicine, you start by practicing what you have just learned but your more important task is to process the new knowledge that comes out as you are practicing. You will be bombarded constantly with information about new drugs, new treatment methods, new bugs, new diseases and new diagnostic tests. If you lag behind in this task, your medical practice will become obsolete even before you notice it and you may have already harmed a patient by prescribing improper treatment.

Chapter 11: Does faith matter?

If you ask the question, "Does grandma's chicken soup really work for cold?", you would get several different answers from different people. You will certainly find a fraction of people for whom it really works. If we analyze the common factor in the group of people for whom it works, we will find that they all firmly believe and have complete faith in that regimen.

You may have also heard about miracles. They happen every now and then in different parts of the world. They happen in all cultures, all religions. Once in a while you hear about sacred

> We hear about miracles all the time. They happen in all cultures, all religions and all parts of the world. But miracles normally only happen to people who believe in them.

water that can cure illness and holy dust that can decrease pain. Again, if you explore these events in detail, one common theme will be identified. They do not work for all. They only work for those who have complete faith in them. Those who drink the water believing that it is holy and it cures their pain, it actually does. But the result is not so certain in those who do not have complete faith in it.

You may be wondering, "What does modern medicine has to do with these mythological stories?"

You may be surprised to hear that this phenomenon is actually widely accepted and well known in modern medicine. When you take anything and firmly and truly believe from the bottom of your heart that this thing will cure your pain, you will be surprised to know that it actually cures you pain. This quality is well described and is called the "placebo effect". It is so important that any clinical research in medicine is invalid if they do not account for the placebo effect.

When a new medicine or a new treatment goes into clinical trial, they always compare it with placebo. Let's say, they have developed a new medicine for back pain and they want to try it on real patients to see how effective it is. When it is about time to test it on real patients, they secretly divide the group of patients who are participating in the trial into two groups. In a good clinical trial, no one knows which patient is in which group, not the doctors and not the patients themselves. One group will receive the new medicine; one will receive the so called "placebo". What is it? It is just an inactive substance or a "sugar pill" that is manufactured to look and test exactly likes the new medicine that is being tested. It is made to let the patients believe that they are getting new medicines. Whenever they analyze the results of that trial, one thing will almost always be true. There will be important improvement in patient's symptoms in both groups. The group of patients that took the inactive fake pills will have measurable improvement in their symptoms.

How do you explain that?

These patients were deliberately deceived during the coarse of the trial. They firmly believed that they were taking this new generation wonder drug that would take their pain away. They had no idea that they were getting fake medicines. It was their strong faith that helped them despite getting the fake medicines.

So, what about the group that actually received the real medicine?

This group also believed that they were getting the new wonder drug that would relieve their suffering. The main difference was that they were ,in fact, getting it unlike the first group. By virtue of the faith itself, this group should have equal amount of pain relief as compared to the first group. By the same logic, they should have additional pain relief if the medicines themselves worked.

This is the exact logic actually applied behind every clinical trial. The group of patients who received the actual treatment should have significantly more pain relief than that could be explained by faith alone. In other words, faith always relieves the pain, new medicine may or may not. They will find that out at the end of the trial.

Lets look at it in a different way. If we did not take into account this "placebo effect", every single medicine in the world would appear to work. All you need is people who believe in them. This effect can be very powerful and effective and is universally accepted.

The placebo effect also demonstrates an interesting aspect of how human body works. It shows the power of your mind over your body. It seems like your mind actually has an ability to heal your body. Otherwise, how do you explain this universally accepted and measurable effect? When you firmly believe that something is good for you, your mind seems to produce some kind of signal in a way that your body actually gets better.

Does this discussion prove that the holy water or the holy dust were just made belief "placebo" effects?

No, it does not. The only way to find out if it actually works is to compare it with placebo. You have to secretly change someone's holy water and substitute it with tap water without that person knowing about it. You have to do it in half of the believers and let the other half keep their holy water. Then you have to compare these two groups of believers and find out if they have any difference in the amount of suffering that has been relieved. So far I have not heard or seen anyone doing this kind of experiment. And until I get that report, I can not make any claims that the holy water is just a placebo effect.

Now, the bigger question is:"When we certainly know that placebo effect is so real and so powerful, why don't we use it in modern medicine?"

In modern medicine, it is unethical. It is unethical to prescribe any medication when it is known that it only works as a placebo.

When you are talking about a disease or condition for which there has been clinical trials that have compared the placebo effect with the real medicine and the real medicine works better, it seems reasonable to think that using the placebo should be unethical. Also using placebo effect on a patient is the moral equivalent of deceiving your patient.

Not all diseases and conditions have known treatment that have been rigorously evaluated in randomized controlled standard clinical trials. Many of these treatment options are continued to be used based on " traditional teaching". "Traditional teaching" in modern medicine is defined as those treatment methods that have been used for a long time and are assumed to work based on what we know about the drug and and the disease. These have never been compared to placebo in a trial.

Traditional teaching is in contrast with the evidence based medicine which is actually a new term that has been used only in the last twenty years. Evidence based medicine actually attempts to compare all treatments with placebo in the clinical trial.

Before the widespread use of evidence based medicine, almost all treatments were based on the anticipated effects of the drugs rather than actual comparison and measurement of the effects in real patients. The scientific knowledge for the anticipation of drug effects were basically obtained from pure medical science. Microbiology, organic chemistry, biochemistry, pathology, physiology and anatomy are examples of branches of medical science that can be classified as pure science as they are composed of rigorous factual data and pure scientific methods as opposed to the art and human factors of clinical medicine. These branches of medical science explore the structure, composition, chemical reactions and biochemical pathways of the human body and explore how different chemical and biochemical elements alter the function of different organ systems of the human body. New drugs were invented and used for the treatment of diseases and conditions based on their known ability to alter certain organ system in a certain way. As these drugs and treatments were based on pure science, they did work as they were predicted to; they had predictable effects on organ systems and altered or modified body chemicals in a certain way. This was the predominant scientific method of modern medicine until about two decades ago. It was gradually noticed over centuries by physicians that although the effect on organ systems and chemical composition of the body by these drugs were predictable, their desired effect on the actual human patient were quite variable.

With the rapid growth in the technology used in modern medicine, many new and innovative drugs and techniques were discovered to alter disease process at the organ level. With this advancement, the difference between drug effect on organs and drug effect on human patients became more apparent. This led to the concept of "evidence based medicine". Evidence based medicine seeks evidence of actual beneficial effects of the drug on the real patient rather than just lab based experiments and scientific predictions. The gold standard or the best evidence comes from clinical trials that are "placebo-controlled double blinded randomized controlled clinical trial".

If we explore why placebo-controlled, double blinded, randomized controlled trials are the gold standard for evidence based medicine, we will find some very interesting aspects of how the human element plays a big role in medical practice. Placebo-controlled means that the drug is being compared with a placebo. Some patients will receive the treatment drug while others will receive a fake pill that looks and smells exactly like the treatment drug. The patients will not know if they are receiving the drug or the inactive substance. Not only the patients, but the doctors and other research staff also do not know which patients are getting drugs and which ones are getting the placebo. This is why it is called double blinded trail.

You probably understand the reason for blinding the patients. You have to make them think that they are all getting the new medication. But, why blind the doctors and the researchers?

It seems like the placebo effect also applies to the doctor giving the medicine. When a doctor believes that the medicine that he is giving to the patient will help the patient, it actually does. When the doctor believes that the medicine works, he will anticipate better outcome in this patient which will probably be reflected in his behavior towards this patient. This in turn will make the patient feel that she is being well cared for. When the patient believes that she is being well cared for by the doctor, this faith could make her better. To avoid any conscious or unconscious difference in the doctor's behavior to the patients in the placebo and the treatment group, it is necessary to blind the doctors as well.

This information is kept top secret until the end of trial. Randomized controlled means that the drugs and placebo are distributed like lottery tickets, any patient can get either the drug or the placebo totally based on her luck.

Patients receiving only the placebo will have some beneficial effects. The trial drug is believed to work only when the beneficial effect is significantly different or higher than those only receiving placebo. In other word, if you did not have a comparison group and wanted to see if a medicine works, you will find out that every single medicine you test would seem to work. When there is no placebo to compare, your trial medicine in itself is working as placebo.

In retrospect, looking at how treatments were decided before evidence based medicine was widely accepted, we can not help but wonder how many of the treatments were merely working as placebo. The physicians who prescribe these drugs believed that these medicine worked based on the scientific reasoning. The patients believed that they worked because they believed in their doctors. The end result was that they actually did work. They only question that remains is:"Were they working as placebo or as actual treatment drug?" This question will remain unanswered until they actually compare that drug with a placebo in a randomized controlled double blinded clinical trial.

But now, we have the answer to one question that was previously raised. If placebo works, why don't we use it in clinical practice? We are using it and it works but the only thing is we do not know when we are using it. If we knew, we would use the real drug instead of placebo. By definition, real treatment regimens tested by gold standard are better than placebo.

Chapter 12: Should not all the doctors treat the same disease same way?

It only seems logical. After all they are the experts in treating diseases and you would expect them to agree on how to treat a particular disease. It may therefore surprise you to learn that doctors do not always agree on how to treat a particular disease.

There are so many different practice variations that, usually, if two patients with exactly same disease go to two different doctors, they will most likely be treated in a slightly different way at each doctor's place. This practice variation exists at different levels. There are individual practice variations even in the same group of doctors working at the same clinic. There are also group variations how certain medical groups practice slightly differently from other medical groups. There is sub-specialty and specialty variation where the practice is slightly different based on which type of specialists treat the same disease. There is community variation where same disease is treated slightly differently based on whether is an urban, suburban or rural community setting. The exact treatment also differs based on whether it is an academic teaching hospital or a community based private practice hospital. If there is so much variation in the treatment pattern, it is only natural that you begin to worry if your doctor is treating you the right way. And if doctors themselves do not agree with each other, how can they expect you to agree with their treatment recommendations?

These are all valid concerns and very good questions. These types of questions are not that easy to answer and explain. Let me try my best in this chapter.

You probably know by now(chapter 10) that medical knowledge keeps evolving with time. The doctor who just graduated from a medical school was taught slightly different material in comparison to the doctor who graduated five years ago. This way, even the basic textbook medical knowledge the particular doctor gained in the medical school differs slightly based on the years since graduation.

After years of graduations, physicians all try to remain current with the medical knowledge by subscribing to different medical journals and professional societies. But the way the new knowledge is acquired and the pace with which it is assimilated into day to day clinical practice is different based on what type of setting the practice is located in. On one extreme, we can look at the university setting inside a teaching hospital. Here medical students, clinical instructors, researchers and professors are avidly searching for new medical information every single day. They are finding, presenting, discussing these new information as they become available within hours or days of first reporting. In a teaching hospital, they are required to explore and extensively review all major new research articles that are published in the medical journals. They all have to reflect everyday on how that new finding may change their understanding of a particular disease and how they might have to change their practice pattern based on that new information. In other words, the doctor who primarily practices in a teaching hospital is mostly current with day to day medical advances.

Hold on a minute. If you were about to close the book and pick up the phone to fire your doctor from the community private practice clinic, please wait until you finish reading this whole chapter. Then you can make an informed decision. It is natural that you would like to be treated by a doctor whose knowledge is as current as possible: current to the day, current to the hour and current to the minute. But does being current to the minute always mean better care?

Teaching hospitals and university hospitals are the places

where they attempt to practice cutting edge medical care. It also means that they are the ones to start the newest treatment as they become available. In most instances, it is a good thing to have the latest form of treatment available with the promise of better treatment outcomes and less side effects. But at the same time, the cutting edge technology can be a double edged sword.

Newest and most advanced treatments also mean that they are not time tested. Usually by the time a new treatment method is published and approved for practice, it has gone through several phases of clinical trial and has been found to be safe for clinical use. But that is not the same thing as being around for a few years and having been widely used in practice all over the county and all over the world. You must have heard on the news now and then that certain medication that was thought to be safe and effective had to be taken off the market as certain harmful effects

> The exact treatment or the exact medication you receive from your doctor not only depends on your disease but also depends on what type of setting the medical practice is located in.

were found after first few years of its use in the real world. In fact, there are far more examples of such cases that do not always make it to the headline news in the mainstream media. There are instances where the new drug is found to be not as good as the older drugs. There are instances when the new treatment did not make as big an impact on the prevention of certain disease as was initially thought. When the impact and effects are not very alarming, it will only be discussed in the medical circle and will not make it to the community.

In summary, if you get your medical care in a university teaching hospital, you will have the opportunity to enjoy the latest medical technology but at the same time, the treatment you receive may not be as time tested and safe as it would be in the real world.

Let's look at the other extreme. Let's say you are from a small rural community and have been going to the same family doctor for the last thirty years and he is the only doctor you know. Your doctor will naturally be somewhat skeptical to the latest treatment or latest technology. He has probably seen a few times in his career where "the latest breakthrough" later proved to be not that great at all. He is therefore not very excited when a new treatment gets reported in the medical journal that he subscribes to every month. Yet, he does keep a subscription to a few essential major medical journals and goes through them about once or twice a month to see what is going on out there. He is definitely not as excited as the young doctor in the university hospital who first read about the treatment two months ago even before it was in the printed journal. Perhaps that young doctor was even following that clinical research even before they announced the results.

But to the rural doctor, it is not that exiting and not that important. He likes to practice time tested methods and the ones that he has been practicing for years. But he too will eventually start using the new method once it starts getting wider acceptance into everyone's clinical practice. It may take a few years for him to start using the new drug that only took a few days for the doctor at the university. You will receive your old time tested and safe medicine from him but you may not get the latest treatment that might have resulted in a better outcome.

In actual practice, every doctor is somewhere in between the two extremes of practice patterns that you just learned. Everyone is assimilating and using new information but at a slightly different pace. It not only depends on the setting of the practice but also on the personality and personal comfort level of the particular physician. But what is more important is that good physicians are always practicing what they believe is the best treatment option for the patient under the circumstances.

Chapter 13: I really fainted. They can not find anything wrong with me.

I am really worried.

Don't worry, you are lucky. I would be worried if they found the reason for your fainting.

Sounds odd? It is true. In medicine, sometimes you are far better off if they do not find any diagnosis for you. The most common example is in the case of fainting. You have probably seen people faint under different circumstances. You might have seen someone faint in a crowded stadium on a hot day. You might have seen someone faint at a concert. You might have seen an anxious speaker faint at the podium. There can also be more serious types of fainting like, a heart patient fainting on his treadmill, or a diabetic patient fainting with dehydration.

Whenever someone faints, some type of medical attention will be sought. In a few cases when the patient is young and healthy and has an obvious reason for fainting that even a lay person can recognize, the patient will be sent home with reassurance. Most of the other patients will likely be kept in the hospital overnight for observation.

This can be very anxiety provoking and difficult time for the patient and the family. The only wish the patient and her family will have is that somehow the doctors will find out what caused her fainting. They are always hoping and praying to get a diagnosis as soon as possible. The loved ones will be visiting the patient anxiously waiting to hear about all the blood tests, x-rays and EKG readings hoping that they could find something and have some answers about why exactly she fainted.

Most of the times hours go by without any answer. She is

only told that they still need to run some more tests and probably have an answer by the next morning. The next morning comes and it is now time for the doctor to round on the patient.

The family asks: "Doctor, what caused her to faint?"

Doctor: "Well, we ran a lot of tests on her. Her blood pressure is normal. Her heart rhythm seems OK. Her EKG and x-rays are all normal."

"Then what caused her to faint?"

"We are not exactly sure but...."

The whole family is disappointed and has lost interest in what else the doctor has to say. They quietly go home but can not help having bad feeling about the whole incident. They start having doubts about the hospital, about the doctor and about modern medicine as a whole.

"How can they tell me that everything is normal when she actually fainted? How could they not find anything with all those tests? Do they not believe that she actually fainted?"

What they do not understand is how lucky she is. Yes, she is very lucky. She is very lucky that the doctor could not find any reason for her fainting.

At the beginning of the chapter, I gave some hints that fainting can be from something as simple as getting too tired, getting too anxious or getting too excited. At the same time, it could be from a very serious condition. It could be the first sign of a severe heart disease or it could be the manifestation of severe diabetes.

Based on the information readily available at the time of initial evaluation, doctors have to make a decision. If it seems obvious that it is a situational type fainting, no complicated tests are done and patients are usually discharged home from the emergency room. They will be reassured that everything is fine and that this is a situational fainting. They will be told not to worry about it.

I really fainted. They can not find anything wrong with me.

Then, there are patients at the other extreme who definitely have signs and symptoms of serious underlying disease. That includes the patient who is having an acute heart attack and has fainted because of that. That includes the patient that has serious bleeding internally and has significant loss of blood resulting in the fainting. These types of fainting could be easy to diagnose quickly in the emergency department and there would not be many unanswered questions.

The only types of fainting in which there are questions and uncertainties are the ones that fall in between the two extremes. These patients are the ones who might just be fine but there is some doubt and the doctor needs to do more tests to be sure. That is the reason these patients will be kept in the hospital for overnight observation and will have a series of regular blood tests and heart tests done to make sure there is no obvious immediately life threatening condition that requires urgent attention. In a small fraction of these patients, there will be some abnormality that will be discovered during these tests and those will be addressed in an urgent manner.

> Doctors can not always find the exact cause of all symptoms. Most of the times when the symptoms can not be explained after multiple diagnostic tests, it actually means that most of the bad and life threatening things have been excluded. But this can be very difficult to explain to a patient who is very anxious to get a diagnosis from the doctor.

In the majority of the patients, no abnormality will be detected and they will be sent home. These patients are lucky that they did not have any serious medical problem. The reason for their fainting was not identified but no bad news was discovered. The doctor is happy and reassured that no diagnosis was made. Any major diagnosis that can explain the fainting is always a bad news. I would be really worried if they found a reason for your fainting.

This concept is somewhat difficult to understand if you are not in the medical profession. When you go to the doctor, you want the doctor to find out what is going on with you. But your doctor is not always able to find out the cause of your symptoms. Let us explore how the doctor normally thinks in a case like that.

Despite all the advancement in diagnostic technology, the doctor can not explain all symptoms. He is, in fact, not always concerned about trying to explain the cause of every symptom. He thinks about a diagnosis when he sees a pattern of symptoms in the right setting that fits with a known pattern of a disease. When the symptoms do not fit any known pattern, his major concern is normally to make sure that it is not one of the bad things that need immediate attention. In other words, his attention will be focused not on finding out what it is but in finding out what it is not.

For example, when the doctor evaluates a patient that has a chest pain which does not fit with any particular disease that can cause chest pain, he is not very interested to find out what it is. His major concern would be to make sure that it is not a heart attack or a blood clot that is presenting in an atypical manner. This concept is sometimes referred to as a "rule out diagnosis". For example, the diagnosis given to this patient at the time would be "rule out heart attack". When all tests are normal and the doctor does not have a reasonable doubt that this could still be a heart attack, then the diagnosis is ruled out.

"I am not sure what caused your chest pain but I am reasonably confidant now that it does not seem like a heart attack."

This is exactly what the doctor can say if he wants to be honest with the patient.

Chapter 14: I do not really want to go to teaching hospitals.

I do not want to be seen by student doctors.

Well, I can understand your concern. Now, let's find what happens in a teaching hospital and who might be seeing you.

Not all the "student doctors" in a teaching hospital are medical students. Some of them are actually doctors undergoing a very advanced training in a very specific area. And there are also several different categories of medical students.

Let's start with the most basic medical student. This is your typical idea of what a medical student is like. He is your third year medical student. He is just starting his clinical rotation. Depending on what time of year it is, he might have seen a few patients but overall he is fairly new to seeing actual patients. He has just had the book knowledge of medicine but does not have much practical knowledge yet. Do not be surprised if he appears a little bit nervous. He is nervous. He is just trying to hide his nervousness from you. He will typically spend a little longer time with you. He seems to be very keen on everything you say and you will find him writing down and making notes of everything you say. In most US hospitals, the medical students normally wear white coats which are only half in length. This might make it easier for you to understand who I am talking about.

Do not be scared if you find this person coming to see you the next time you are in the hospital. Do not worry, his lack of practical knowledge or his inexperience will not cause any harm to you. That is because, most of the time, he will have very little or no say in the final decision about your diagnosis and treatment. In other words, he is at the bottom of the food chain. He is only allowed to convey your story and your situation to his seniors. He is not allowed to make any decision by himself and he is not even allowed to give you any specific recommendation without consulting with his seniors.

So, he is basically useless to you, isn't he? Is he a complete a waste of you time?

Now, you might say "I told you so, that is why I do not want to go to these teaching hospitals."

On the contrary, he could be your great resource. The one thing that he has that his seniors do not have is time. He has plenty of time to spend with you as he is only assigned a small number of patients as compared to his seniors.

How will that benefit you? Well, you can talk to him about anything. You could explore different possible diagnosis with him. You can give him details that his seniors might not have time to listen to. Also, you can ask him as many questions as you may have. You can even ask him general health questions that you may have, even ones that are not related to your current diagnosis.

Do not underestimate the depth of medical knowledge that the third year medical student has. It is not the medical knowledge that he lacks, it is the real life experience. And exactly because he lacks real life experience, he tends to do everything by the book. That is why it takes him so long to go through everything. He is actually checking things off of his check list- one by one. One benefit of doing things with a check list and going by the book is that his methods are very thorough. He is not jumping to conclusions early and he is not focusing on the common scenario based on experience as he simply does not have any experience at all. As a result, there are always stories of how a smart medical student occasionally made a diagnosis that everyone else had overlooked. It is not because he is smarter than the real doctors but because he has to use the very basic methodological and meticulous ways to arrive at his conclusion.

The minds of an experienced physician has normally been pre-programmed to recognize certain patterns based on experience. He cannot help but reach a conclusion in his mind about your problem just by processing the most obvious information. He has seen similar cases many many times during his practice. But to the medical student, he has to put everything together one by one in place to be able to draw any "big picture" in his mind.

The next level of medical student that you might encounter is the fourth year medical student. He looks about the same as the third year medical student. He has the same type of white coat but appears more confident and less nervous. He has at least one year of experience dealing with the real patients but is still in the medical school and is not a licensed doctor yet. He still cannot make any major decision on his own and has to consult his seniors before he writes any order in your chart. His orders still

> Not all student doctors that you meet in a teaching hospital are medical students. You will have medical students, interns, residents and fellows that are in several different stages of their medical training. Some of them are fully licensed doctors.

have to be co-signed by his supervising doctor before they can be taken by the nurses. But unlike the third year student, he is expected to make his own diagnostic and treatment plans and discuss that with his supervising doctors. Although the final decision will only be made by the supervising doctor, he does have some input in your treatment plan. After all, by the end of that year, he will be getting his medical degree.

The benefit of having the fourth year medical student in your care is almost similar to having a third year medical student. You do not have to worry about being seen by the fourth year student because you will still be independently seen by a licensed physician before any major treatment plans are made. These fourth year medical students are sometimes also called sub-interns or sub-I's in the short because they will be in their internship next year — the year after they graduate.

In most states, after he graduates from medical school, he does not automatically get the license to practice medicine. He has to go into the formal post-graduate training program called "residency". This is the training where he chooses one of the several major branches of medical practice. During his residency training, the resident doctors can legally practice medicine but can only do so in the supervision of another fully licensed doctor. The first year of this residency training is called the internship. If you see an over-worked, tired looking doctor who is running all over the hospital all the time, then that might be your intern. He is normally the one that usually comes in very early in the morning and wakes you up. He still seems a little nervous but appears much more confident than the medical students. He also seems to ask you a lot of questions but his questions seem to be more structured and organized. He does seem to spend enough time with you but his time seems more structured and you will soon notice that he does not have the almost unlimited time that your medical students had.

He can and will write medications for you and his orders do not have to be co-signed by anyone else. He can make many urgent and pressing medical decisions on the spot without consulting anyone. But for the most part, he still has to discuss his plans with and get an OK from his seniors before any major decisions are made. Also, he seems to be spending a whole lot of time in front of the nursing desk as he is the main link between the rest of the doctors and the nursing staff. He, not only has to talk to you and examine you to get information from you, but also has to talk to the nurses and make note about the information the nurses have gathered about you. He is always acting as the middle man between his seniors and the nurses. He gets information from the nurses. He puts that information together and presents it systematically to his supervisor and they will discuss the plan of care and will make a treatment decision. Again, it is his job to communicate with the nurses about the final treatment plans.

I do not really want to go to teaching hospitals.

He is able to answer most of your questions with confidence, especially, if he has already discussed the case with his supervisors. He will be getting more confident making medical decision by the end of the year. Normally, when he starts in July, he seems to say: "I will discuss this with my seniors and get back to you." But if you happen to meet him in June, he is answering your questions with confidence. He has to. The next month in July, he will become a second year resident and he will be supervising the fresh new interns that arrive to the hospital.

Now the next category of in-training doctors you meet are the second and third year residents. For the most part, the second and the third year residents will be appearing very similar to you and you may not be able to tell the difference at all. They behave almost like the interns but are much more confident and seem to be very independent. You will mostly see them with the interns. They seem to be guiding and instructing and checking on the interns all the time. They have to because anything the intern does has to be agreed upon by the senior resident. And the senior resident's duty is to make sure the interns are doing their jobs properly.

Now, who do the residents report to? They report to your attending physicians. These are the top dogs. They are on the top of the food chain. The buck stops with them. Well, in a teaching hospital, they appear to be the highest authority but in fact, they are just your regular doctors. They have been through their medical school, internship and residency and now they are fully licensed to practice medicine independently. These are the doctors you normally see surrounded by a group of young doctors. They seem to be always giving instructions and orders to the residents and interns. Well, they are the doctors that are directly and legally responsible for your care.

All the information collected by the nurses, the interns, the medical students, and the residents finally go to him. He usually does not have to spend a lot of time with you because by the time he is seeing you, he has already collected all the information from everyone else that has seen you so far. So, when he visits you, he is basically rechecking the facts to make sure he is getting the correct information. He will be summarizing the care plan that has already been discussed with you and he will be answering any further questions about your care that you may still have.

Well, so for you have learned about the third year medical student, the fourth year medical student or the sub-I, the first year resident or the intern, the second and higher year resident or the resident proper, and finally the attending physician.

Now there will be another category of in-training doctors involved in your care in a teaching hospital. They are called fellows.

A fellow is the doctor who has finished his residency training and is pursuing further specialization to go into one of the more specialized branches of medical practice. A heart specialist has to do fellowship in Cardiology. A lung specialist has to do fellowship in Pulmonology. He is a licensed fully independent practitioner but still follows directions from his attending physician who is a sub-specialist himself. He is the one who appears very ambitious and sharp and has a lot of confidence. You will normally meet him only if you have a sub-specialist involved in your care. When they need a heart doctor right away, he will be the one to respond first. After he sees you and you need a major heart procedure done, he will come back to you with the attending cardiologist with him. When he finishes his training, he will become an attending cardiologist himself.

Chapter 15: I have been taking this medicine for a long time.

I do not feel any better at all, should I stop?

You may be surprised to know that not all medicines are designed to make you feel better. Yes, that is true. These medications are not meant to improve your symptoms at all. You will not notice any visible change or any relief of any problems with these medications. You must be wondering what these medications are and why are they prescribed at all if they do not make you feel any better.

> Some medicines are not designed to make you feel better. They do not help with with your symptoms at all but are beneficial in the long term. These are actually the medications that are prescribed most frequently in the United States.

You may be surprised to know that these are actually the kind of medications that are prescribed most frequently in the United States. Most of the medical regimen prescribed for chronic asymptomatic medical problems fall into this category. Do not worry, I am going to explain what chronic asymptomatic medical problems mean.

Based on time course of a disease, they can be separated into two broad categories. Acute and chronic. The word "acute" sounds like this may be the more severe form of the disease. But, in reality, the acute or chronic nature of a disease does not have anything to do with the seriousness or severity of the disease. Acute disease or illness is one which has a short time course. It can be a life threatening severe disease or just a minor inconvenience but it has a short onset and short duration.

Example of a minor acute condition is acute upper respiratory infection which is another way of describing common cold. Acute viral gastroenteritis or simply "stomach flu" is another example of an acute disease process. Acute myocardial infarction or a "heart attack" is another acute disease process but can be life threatening. Acute appendicitis is another disease that has a very short course but can be life threatening without immediate surgery.

In the same way, chronic medical illness includes diseases and processes that can be minor or major and life threatening. But all of them have one thing in common. They have a long time course that is measured in months and years instead of days. One example of a disease that is very serious and potentially life threatening but has a long duration is HIV infection. The other similar disease is chronic hepatitis C infection which can also be deadly but has a very long duration of disease course. Chronic disease that is mild and not life threatening is exemplified by chronic osteoarthritis or joint pain that goes on for many many years.

Among these chronic diseases (both severe and mild) there are certain diseases that give you symptoms or problems that you can feel during the whole course of the disease. But there are certain other diseases that remain silent throughout their course until they have reached the final stage of the disease course.

These types of diseases that have a long silent phase are not discovered by the patient but are diagnosed by the doctor based on physical exam and lab tests. The patient does not have any symptom in the early silent phase. Despite being silent, these diseases are not inactive. They are very active inside the your body but do not give you any symptom until it is too late. The most common example of this type of disease is hypertension or high blood pressure.

Hypertension in itself does not cause any symptom in the silent phase but can continue to damage your internal body organs and you will only have symptoms when one of the organs is damaged. It Is therefore also called "silent killer". Most of the times high blood pressure is diagnosed during a routine doctor visit but it could also be discovered when seeking medical attention for other unrelated medical problem.

If the patient initially sought medical attention for other unrelated symptoms, she will likely be called back to follow up on the the blood pressure to check it again. If it is still high, she will be started on medication for "treatment" of the hypertension. This patient will most likely need to be on medication for hypertension for a very long time. But the patient did not have any symptom from the hypertension to begin with. It is therefore very unlikely that the patient would feel any better by being on the medicine. These types of medicines help prevent complication and organ system damage from a chronic medical problem. But you are not supposed to feel any better or any worse after taking that medicine.

I am sure you have definitely met a lot of people who feel much better after they started taking the medications for hypertension. How do you explain that?

It is relatively easy to explain. They are the people who believed that the blood pressure medicine that the doctor gave them will make them feel better. If you read chapter 11, you know that if people take something and have complete faith in it, they will actually feel better even if they were taking fake medicines. It is, therefore, only natural that they feel better taking these pills but these pills are designed to control their blood pressure and help prevent complications, not designed to help with their symptoms.

There are many different categories of medicines in this class that are all designed to prevent complications and bad outcomes but not designed to help with any symptom. Medications for high blood pressure, medications for high cholesterol, medications to prevent stroke, medications to prevent blood clots and medications to prevent heart attacks are a few examples of medications that will not help you feel any better after you take them.

After reading about all these medications that are designed to prevent heart attacks and strokes, you might question: "If we have so many medications to prevent heart attacks and strokes, why do people still get heart attacks and strokes?"

You may think that heart attacks and strokes happen to people who are not taking these preventive medications. But that is wrong. People who are taking these medications still can have heart attacks and strokes.

In fact, you will find people who are doing everything to prevent stroke but still end up having stroke. They take medications to prevent stroke, they do regular physical activity, they watch what they eat, they maintain a healthy weight, they follow all the directions from their doctors, they get their cholesterol checked as recommended by their doctor and take cholesterol medications if needed. But some of them still end up having strokes anyway.

But how could this happen? Whose fault is that? Is it a failure of modern medicine?

Before we answer these questions, we need to find out how disease prevention works.

The first step to find out how to prevent a disease is to find out what causes the disease in the first place. You need to find out the mechanisms of the disease. Unlike modern clinical medicine, the actual biological science of medicine is very advanced. The scientific knowledge about the mechanisms of diseases is very advanced and very detailed. They have explored these mechanisms to minute details going from the organ level to cellular level and even to molecular level. Let's talk about these two disease processes that we just mentioned — heart attack and stroke. Let us try to explore the cause of these diseases.

If you simply ask:"What causes a heart attack and a

stroke?"

The simple answer is: "It is the loss of blood supply to these organs that causes the heart attack and the stroke. If the blood supply to the heart is blocked, it causes a heart attack. If the blood supply to a part of the brain is blocked, it causes a stroke."

"Are you sure?"

"Yes, we are sure. This has been looked at biologically and scientifically. We are completely sure."

As highly scientific and definite this answer is, you cannot help but ask further questions in this case: "Then what causes the blood supply to be blocked?"

"Well most of the times, it is the disease of the blood vessel that supplies blood to the organ.",simple enough.

Again another question follows naturally.

"So, what could happen to the blood vessel that can cause them to be blocked?"

This time the answer would be a little bit more complex.

"It could be a number of things but the most common is the formation of a clot that blocks that artery."

Again another question follows:"Then, what causes the formation of that clot?"

The answer gets even more complicated by now.

"There are small particles in the blood that are called platelets, they stick together and form a clot."

Now, whether you understand about platelets or not, you will definitely have another question ready.

"Then what causes the platelets to stick together?"

It is getting even more complicated now. Now the answers are getting less definitive and more general.

"It could be a number of different causes. It could be a defect of the platelets. It could be because of a plaque build-up on the artery. It could also be because of blood being too thick."

Now you can still ask more questions but you have to pick and choose one of the many causes to ask what causes that.

In this case you can pick one and ask:"Then what causes the plaque built-up in the artery?"

The answer could be:"It could be a number of different causes such as high cholesterol, smoking, hereditary factors, age, immune system problem etc."

With this answer, we are effectively moving from the factual knowledge of basic biological science into the less certain area of clinical medicine. Now you can see how it is difficult to prevent a heart attack by just using a pure biological reasoning. We clearly understand how a heart attack happens inside a human body and can also explain the chain of biological events leading to it. But each step in the chain of events have different possible causes and when you trace the individual cause and try to find its cause, it finally ends up in some outside factor, environmental factor (smoking), hereditary factor (family history of similar problems), or lifestyle factors (lack of exercise) etc. When it gets to this level, it becomes very difficult to explain things with scientific accuracy as these things can not be tested in a lab.

You can test the blood of a person who smokes cigarettes in the lab and compare it to the blood from a person who does not smoke cigarettes but you will not be able to tell if the difference is just because of the smoking or because of other factors such as lifestyle, family medical history, diet etc. At this stage, we can only infer what factors play a role in increasing the chance of a heart attack but cannot definitely and scientifically prove it by lab experiment or simple reasoning. There are many things that are known to increase the risk of a heart attack but not all of them can be controlled or reversed. By decreasing and modifying some of these known possible causes of heart attack, you can decrease the chances of having one but the risk will never go down to zero.

Now, you may ask:"What about the drug advertised on TV? They show an impressive animation of how the clot is formed by the platelets and how that particular medicine keeps blood platelets from sticking together and forming clots. They even tell you to ask your doctor about that medicine."

That is a very effective way of marketing that drug that makes it seem like as long as you are taking that medication, you do not have to worry about a heart attack at all.

Yes, it does reduce one cause of a particular step in a certain type of heart attack but it is not as simple as shown in the animation. If it were completely true, no one taking that medicine should ever have a heart attack and that is not true. Remember increased stickiness of the platelets is only one of the causes of clot formation and clot formation in the blood vessel is only one of the causes of a blocked artery. And again, an artery blocked by a clot is only one of the many causes of heart attacks.

At the same time, this drug makes platelets less sticky not completely non-sticky.

Well, you may ask, "Why don't they make a drug that makes these platelets completely non-sticky?"

To answer that:"That drug would be a very effective poison."

Yes, if they make a drug that completely prevents the platelets from sticking together, that drug would easily kill you. If the platelets cannot stick together at all, they wont be able to plug any holes in your blood vessels at all. If you scratch yourself or even rub your skin or brush your tooth, you will puncture a small blood vessel. Once punctured, the bleeding will not stop because the platelets are completely non-sticky and cannot plug the hole and the result would be that you could bleed to death. Therefore any drug designed to prevent platelets from forming a clot should be designed in a way that it prevents a large clot to prevent a heart attack but still allows small clots to form to prevent bleeding.

As we move our discussion from the artery, platelets and blood clots to heart attacks, lifestyle, smoking and hereditary factors, we are loosing the ability to conduct lab experiments to test our theories. Then, how do we find out how to prevent heart attacks?

We can do clinical trials to find these answers. You read about some aspects of clinical trial in chapter 11. We will be talking more about them here with a slightly different perspective.

Let's say, we have a new medicine that decreases the stickiness of the platelet to a very good degree where it prevents heart attack without causing major bleed. To prove this, we need to design a clinical trial. We will need two groups of patients. Both groups should be approximately identical in their age and risk factors for heart disease. If we are testing this kind of a strong drug, we will probably have to test it in patients with very high risks of heart attack such as patients that already had at least one heart attack in the past. Then we randomly assign these patients into two groups.

One group will receive all standard treatment plus a fake pill and the other group will receive all standard treatment plus this new medicine. We will then follow these patients closely over a period of time. At the end of the trial, we will count the number of patients who had heart attack during that period of time in both groups. Then, we will make calculations as to which group has less percentage of heart attacks. If the percentage of heart attacks is significantly lower in the new medicine group, we can conclude that the new medicine probably reduces heart attack.

There is one interesting thing that we can note here. Earlier in our discussion, we were talking about patients having heart attacks or strokes despite doing everything to prevent them. We can find good examples of such patients here. If you noticed, these are the patients that were all getting standard treatment for prevention of heart attack. If these preventions were full proof, no one of these patients should have any heart attack. If that drug prevented heart attack just like shown on TV, then no one of these patients would have a heart attack.

But the reality is different. That is why when drug companies make claims about their new medicine, they do not claim that the medicine stops heart attack. They advertise that the new treatment reduces the risk of heart attack by what percentage over standard treatment.

Now let's say the new drug reduces heart attack by 50%. Sounds very impressive, doesn't it? Let's find out what does that mean before you rush to the phone to "call your doctor now" as suggested by the ad.

Let's say, they had 500 patients in each group. The first group had 10 patients with heart attack at the end of the first year. Now let's say that the group with new medicine had 5 patients with heart attack. This makes the percentage of heart attacks in the first group 2% and the percentage of heart attacks in the second group 1%. Now if you take it literally, it means that if two in one hundred had heart attack with the standard treatment, only one in one hundred would have heart attack with the standard treatment plus the new medicine. This literally means that the new drug could save one out of one hundred or 1% more heart attacks over the standard treatment.

But this statement,"The new medicine saves 1 more percentage of heart attack."would not sound very impressive to put it in the promotion of the new drug, would it? Now let's put it in a slightly different way. Lets put it as a ratio instead of the actual difference. From the above discussion, the risk of heart attack was 2% with the standard treatment and was 1% with the standard treatment plus the new drug. Now instead of stating the actual difference, lets put it as a ratio. The actual difference in the rate of the heart attacks was one percent and the rate of heart attack in the standard treatment was two percent. If you divide one by two, you get 50%. Sounds good! Let's report this number instead of the actual difference. This number is called Relative

Risk Reduction and is just a ratio of the two risks, not the actual difference. This is the number the drug companies like to report.

The previous number which was calculated to be 1% is called the Absolute Risk Reduction which is the actual difference between the two risks. This is the number mostly used by academic researchers and clinicians because it is more useful in calculating the actual risks. The Absolute Risk Reduction can also be used to calculate the Number Needed to Treat(NNT). Number Needed to Treat gives you an estimate number of patients you have to treat with this new medicine in order to prevent one heart attack. If you simply divide 1 by the Absolute Risk Reduction number, you get the Number Needed to Treat. Here it is 1 divided by 1% which is equivalent to 100. It means that when you treat 100 new patients with this medicine on top of the standard treatment, you may save one more heart attack.

We have not yet discussed about potential harm from the medication. With a medication that makes your platelets less sticky, the obvious harm that can happen is bleeding. They will also have to look at how many patients in the first group had serious bleeding and how many in the new drug group had it. Then we can calculate the difference in major bleeding risks in these two groups the same way we calculated the heart attack risks. That is why they always tell you to discuss the possible benefits and possible harm from a new treatment with your doctor.

Now you probably understand that doing all the right thing does not mean that you are immune from having these bad diseases. Doing the right thing is very important because it reduces your risk. Taking your regular blood pressure medicine is very important because you can at least control your blood pressure with it. Controlling your blood pressure reduces the risk of having a stroke or a heart attack. It may not make you feel better but makes you less likely to have bad things in the future. But a low risk does not mean that it will not happen. Even if the risk has been down to 1 in a million, there is always that one

I have been taking this medicine for a long time.

unlucky person in one million who will have it. And when it happens to you, it matters 100% to you even though the risk was 1 in a million.

Chapter 16: An interesting case

In medical literature, a case report is a description of a patient encounter that has some significance or importance because of some unusual circumstances. It could be that the particular disease is so rare that they are surprised to have found one. It could also be that the particular patient had a very unusual presentation of a common disease and they were particularly happy to have recognized and diagnosed it properly. Sometimes it could simply be that they tried a new treatment and it seemed to work. But in any circumstance, the reason for publishing that case report is because other doctors are interested to read it and relate to it and could get some education or important information from it. I have written several case reports myself throughout my medical career with the target reader being another doctor.

> Case reports in medical literature are mostly written because other doctors are interested to read them because of some unusual or interesting event. This is my first case report where the target reader is you instead of another doctor.

This will be the first case report where the target reader is you instead of another doctor. In our medical career, we meet and greet people from all walks of life. We do remember most of our patients but the memory is normally very brief. We are only able to recall just a few snippets of their life if we happen to meet them under different circumstances. But there are always exceptions. There are a few patients you remember in details. For that to happen, you must have had an extraordinary event when you were taking care of the patient. Sometimes, it could be a very unexpected bad outcome. At other times, it could be a very surprising and unexpected good outcome. A few times, it could just be a very extraordinary personality of the patient that could have made you think and reflect about yourself and your career. At some other times it could be because of something the patient had was so difficult to diagnose that you had to think about it for days and had to research so much before you were able to reach at the right diagnosis. The case I am going to describe has a little bit of everything that I just described. Obviously, I have not included any personal or identifying information about the patient himself.

A thirty year old male was brought to the ER by the police after they found him completely unresponsive lying on the side of a barn in a summer day. He seemed to be breathing OK and his heart was beating fine but they were not able to get any response from the person at all. He would not speak, not move at all and not even open his eyes.

I went down to the emergency department myself to see the patient after they called me. I decided to go down and see the patient myself before accepting to admit him under my care because the story and the circumstances seemed somewhat unusual to me. I wanted to make sure there was no unusual or emergent condition that was being overlooked.

When I saw the patient, I was completely lost. I could not figure out what was going on with him. I was not able to get any type of response from him and he might have been completely dead except that his heart was beating normally and that he was breathing normally. If you recall chapter 2 and chapter 3, you know that this would be a difficult patient to diagnose because he is not going to tell me what is wrong with him. I was on my own this time.

Now, where do I start? Even under these circumstances, I still needed to get the whole picture. I needed someone to tell me what was wrong with the patient. I decided not to look at any tests or any scans before getting the answer to the question: "Why is he here?" or "Tell me what happened?" As the patient was not able to answer these questions, I decided to ask the person who brought him to the hospital. And that was the police officer sitting outside the patient room guarding him.

Then, I got the bigger picture. Or, at least I thought I did. The police officer told me that they were chasing a car that was involved in a hit and run case. The driver then decided to run from the police and went off speeding violently and had several police cars chasing him. He managed to get into the highway and drove far enough to get out of the city and into the country. By that time they had many police cars looking for him and eventually they were able to close in on him. At that time, he suddenly went off the road and drove his car into a ditch in front of a barn. When the police eventually reached there to look in the car, he was gone. They started ground search for about 25 minutes before they located him. There they found this man in his thirties who seemed completely unconscious but did not have any signs of physical injury. There was not a single bruise in his skin and there was no swelling or bleeding anywhere.

By this time I at least had the answer to the question: "What happened?" Then, I went ahead and reviewed all the blood-work and CAT scans the patient had done in the ER. At least, I knew what to look for. I was looking for things that could make a man in his thirties to become unconscious after a police chase and possible trauma. Several possibilities crossed my mind. The patient could have a blunt head trauma where his head could have been hit by some blunt object that caused internal injury without leaving any superficial wound. Another possibility was that he was acting irrationally and was running from the police, he could have been on some street drugs that could made him behave that way and could also be responsible for his current condition. Another possibility was that he could have some kind of neurological condition that could explain his irrational behavior and unresponsive state. What other possible reasons you can think of ? Yes, that thought crossed my mind too. It was indeed possible that he could have been faking unconsciousness to avoid being arrested and face the legal consequences. But, as physicians, we normally do not let that thought come to the front of our brain unless we have excluded all other possibilities.

Subsequently, I reviewed his blood-work including his toxicology screen which is a blood test to detect common types of street drugs in the system. He did have some traces of marijuana and cocaine in his system. But that failed to explain everything.

Yes, cocaine is a very dangerous drug and it can kill you instantly but the way cocaine kills you is slightly different. Cocaine causes your heart rate and your blood pressure to go so high that it can cause too much pressure can can damage your blood vessels. In other words, it can make your heart beat so fast and so strong that your body can not tolerate it. But his heart rate was normal and his blood pressure was only slightly elevated which is very common in any type of stressful situational. I then reviewed his EKG which is an electric tracing of the heartbeat. EKG is a test designed to detect a heart attack or heart rhythm problems.

His EKG was normal. Does that mean that he did not have a heart attack? If you read chapter 4, you know that the answer is no. It only means that it was less likely to be a heart attack and I had to look for some more likely cause for his condition. Of note, cocaine can cause heart attack and it does so by damaging the the blood vessels that actually supply blood to the heart muscle itself.

Next, I looked at the CAT scan of his head. It appeared pretty normal to me. His brain size seemed to be appropriate for his body and his age. He did not seem to have any bleeding or any stroke in his brain. Of coarse, he could still have one of those bad things. We just had to wait and see.

That's what we did next. We just waited and observed him closely. We hoped he would somehow wake up in the next few hours and I could ask him what really happened. But, that did not happen. In the next few hours, he remained very stable but was still unresponsive. We then went ahead and started giving him fluid and glucose through his veins to support his body system while he is in a state that could be called a "coma". At that time, we started doing some special neurological tests on him. These tests were designed to detect the presence of brain function at different levels of human brain. When we think about the "brain", most people think only about the higher intellectual brain function which is thinking, reading etc. But brain is, in fact, the organ that gives signals to move each and every part of our body. All the muscles in your body follow the commands of your brain. When you brain does not tell your hand to move, it can not move on its own.

There are different tests to see which part of the brain is active and which parts are not. The way to do these tests is to give certain stimulus to the brain and see how it responds. The simplest of such test is to just pinch someone. When you do that, brain senses the pain and responds appropriately. Of course,you would not do that to a person that you know has the pain senses intact. But that test might help you when you are in doubt about the integrity of that patient's sensation of pain. In our patient who was not responding at all to all common stimuli, we had to give him some special stimulus.

I will describe here one such test that is normally done only in patients in a comatose state to determine the depth of the coma and to find out which layers of the brain might be still active. There are different ways of doing this and this is only one of the several methods. You have to be able to watch the movement of the patient's eyeball very closely for this test. In our patient we had to get one person to forcefully open and keep his eyes open during the test to look into his eyeballs. Then, we prepared about half a cup of ice-cold water and injected that water into his left ear while observing closely to see if there would be any eye movement. We finished the test and his eyeballs only had a very tiny movement which we were not able conclude whether that was a positive response or not.

At that time, the previous thought crossed my mind again that this patient might have been faking unconsciousness to get away from the police. But I hoped and prayed that it was not the case because that would have been the worst possible torture if he was awake. As this test is designed to get reaction from even the semi-comatose brain, it is a very strong and very unpleasant sensation which is many times worse than pain and perhaps many times more severe than water-boarding. For that reason we quickly let our scientific brain take control of our emotional brain and stopped thinking it as a form of torture but continued to think of it as an important medical test.

After this test was inconclusive, we went ahead and did more tests. We did MRI of his brain. We did CT scan of his chest. We did ultrasound of his neck blood vessels. We did EEG. We repeated EKG several times. But we could not get any answers.

We then consulted another doctor, a very skilled Neurologist. He reviewed all the tests done by then and went ahead and did a detailed neurological exam of the patient. Again the detailed neurological exam involved the test we just described and also many other different tests that could definitely be classified as torture in an awake patient. The neurologist was also at a complete loss. After repeated testing and all normal tests, he was more forthcoming with the idea that this could represent a case of "psychogenic coma" which is another way of saying that he could have been faking this all the time. The reason he was saying this was because he definitely felt like there was some small eye movement with the test we described earlier. If the patient was completely comatose, he would not have any eye movement at all in response to the test. He then postulated that the fact that his eyes seemed to move just a little bit could mean that he might have been voluntarily suppressing his eye movements. I did think about that possibility but quickly dismissed it as being very unlikely as I thought:"Who could bear such a torture and still manage to not even move the eyeball?" I went out on my own scratching my head trying find other possible cause for his condition.

It was four days since he arrived to the hospital. He was still lying in bed not moving at all. We had already started him on blood thinners to make his blood less susceptible to form blood clots. When people are in bed without moving, the blood starts to pool in the lower part of the body and can form blood clots that can be life threatening.

On the fourth day, I got a call with a very excited voice. It was the nurse taking care of that patient. She told me that the patient suddenly woke up and was asking for food. I ran to his room and started asking him questions. He was in no mood to talk to me. He was just pleading me for some food. After I quickly checked his pulse and his blood pressure, I gave the permission to the nurse to bring him some food. He started eating very fast and only after about ten minutes of eating, he started to talk to me.

He said: "Yes doc, I was completely awake when you did all that nonsense to me. I was just trying to get away from the police. I know I messed up."

I asked him:"If you were able to tolerate that kind of torture and not even blink your eyes, what was it that made you give up everything wake up?"

He said: "I got so hungry that I thought I would die from hunger!"

Of coarse, we were not giving him any food because he seemed to be in a coma. We were giving him water and nutrition through his veins. No, he would not have died from the hunger.

But the nutrition we gave him was only enough to sustain his life. It did nothing to curb his hunger. After this realization, the medical mystery of this case was solved. It was a case of psychogenic coma which is a very rare condition but does happen now and then. Usually these patients have some underlying psychiatric problem that makes them think in a slightly unusual way. These patients have very high tolerance for pain and torture. Otherwise, a normal person would not have been able to fake coma even for an hour.

On that day, I had a bigger realization about humanity and human civilization. It came to my mind that hunger is not only the biggest torture and biggest cause of human suffering but is also the main driving force of human civilization. The cavemen risked their lives and went out for hunting. They developed better hunting tools to find food to cure their hunger. Without hunger, there would have not been such a strong force behind human civilization.

www.ingramcontent.com/pod-product-compliance
Lightning Source LLC
Chambersburg PA
CBHW072233290326
41934CB00008BA/1271
9780982696507